Solving Children's Soiling

For Churchill Livingstone:

Senior Commissioning Editor: Sarena Wolfaard
Project Development Manager: Dinah Thom
Project Manager: Andrea Hill
Design Direction: Judith Wright

Solving Children's Soiling Problems

A Handbook for Health Professionals

Jackie Bracey BSc(Hons) RGN RM SNCert
School Nurse Co-ordinator and Practice Teacher, Nottingham City
Primary Care Trust, Nottingham, UK

Foreword by

June Rogers MBE
Continence Advisor, Paediatric Nurse Advisor (Special Needs),
Prescot Clinic, Prescot, UK

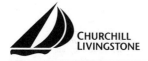

CHURCHILL
LIVINGSTONE

EDINBURGH LONDON NEW YORK PHILADELPHIA ST LOUIS SYDNEY TORONTO 2002

CHURCHILL LIVINGSTONE
An imprint of Elsevier Science Limited

cover photo © imaging-body.com
The right of Jackie Bracey to be identified as the author of this work
has been asserted by her in accordance with the Copyright, Designs
and Patents Act 1988.

First published 2002

ISBN 0 443 07144 6

British Library Cataloguing in Publication Data
A catalogue record for this book is available from the British Library

Library of Congress Cataloging in Publication Data
A catalog record for this book is available from the Library of Congress

Note
Medical knowledge is constantly changing. As new information
becomes available, changes in treatment, procedures, equipment and
the use of drugs become necessary. The author and the publishers have
taken care to ensure that the information given in this text is accurate
and up to date. However, readers are strongly advised to confirm that
the information, especially with regard to drug usage, complies with
the latest legislation and standards of practice.

The
publisher's
policy is to use
**paper manufactured
from sustainable forests**

Printed in China by RDC Group Limited

Contents

Foreword

It is a great privilege to be asked to write the foreword of this book as it covers a common childhood problem that is very dear to my heart. Most of us who work with children with continence problems, particularly those who soil, are aware of the devastating effect this can have on the child and family. However, those practitioners who do not have this 'inside knowledge' often trivialise the problem and fail to address the soiling issues appropriately.

The publication of the Good Practice Guidelines in Continence Care (Department of Health 2000) and the push towards developing more primary care based services provide a climate for change and the opportunity for the development of appropriate nurse-led services. The important role school nurses and health visitors play in providing advice and support for children and their families with toiletting problems is well established. This, therefore, is an ideal time for the development of specific nurse-led services for children with constipation and soiling.

This book will act as a valuable starting point for those involved with children with a soiling problem, and stimulate debate regarding 'best practice'. Each chapter covers a different aspect of the issues involved and is written in a style which makes for easy reading. In addition to the chapters on normal development of bowel control and causes of constipation, there are other chapters on related subjects, including urinalysis and complementary therapies. Examples of charts and assessment forms are also given.

This book gives an excellent overview of managing a child with a soiling problem and offers practical advice regarding treatment interventions. By raising awareness of this childhood problem it may hopefully stimulate others to develop an interest and gain more insight into addressing this distressing condition.

June Rogers MBE

REFERENCE

Department of Health 2000 Good practice in continence services. DoH, London

Preface

Why write a book on soiling? As a school nurse I have long been interested in children's continence. My interest started with enuresis, when I was studying its management and running clinics. After an in-service training course on continence promotion, I designed a training pack aimed at school nurses and health visitors which I later delivered to all the school nursing staff in my unit. I needed a subject for my BSc dissertation, and soiling seemed the next most appropriate area to investigate. I also thought it would enhance the service given to the children on my caseload.

During the literature search for the subject, it became apparent that there was little written information on the management of soiling. I continued to teach other staff about enuresis but now also began to teach about soiling on an in-house children's continence course. During one of these courses, when discussing the lack of a basic text on soiling, a group said jokingly I should write a book about it. Although I dismissed the idea at the time the thought took hold. When I approached the publishers I thought they would commission someone else to write the book. The proposal was accepted and the book was to be written by me! I wanted a text that was easy to read and within most people's price range.

Although this book is aimed at nurses, particularly school nurses and health visitors, I hope that it will appeal to all staff groups that manage children with chronic constipation leading to soiling. The book is designed to be read from front to back, but equally it can be dipped into for information on a specific area.

Nottingham 2002   Jackie Bracey

Acknowledgements

I would like to thank my husband and my son, who have, for many months, accepted the fact that I was hidden away pounding on the computer keyboard while writing this book. They have listened to my frustrations when writer's block struck and my enthusiasm when the book flowed well. My thanks also to my mother and my late father, who always encouraged us to think we could achieve; to colleagues who have listened to me expounding my intentions and have read chapters (sometimes even in bed, to their husbands' disgust) and put up with my, at times, boring theories. Yet they still speak to me! To everyone who has encouraged me to go for it! Here it is.

Abbreviations

BNF	British National Formulary
Ig E	Immunoglobulin E
MIMS	Monthly Index of Medical Specialities
MSU	Mid stream urine
UKCC	United Kingdom Central Council for Nursing, Midwifery and Health Visiting
UTI	Urinary tract infection

1

Introduction

Mention soiling to people and besides the facial expression indicating disgust many will tell you that the child must have a psychological problem. Loening-Baucke (Kamm & Lennard-Jones
1994) tells us, 'It is important to point out that the stooling problem is caused by the underlying constipation and is not caused by
a disturbance in the psychological behaviour of the child.'
Although health professionals working with children who soil
have long recognised that the cause of their patients' problems is
chronic constipation with overflow, this knowledge does not
appear to be widespread. The aim of this book is to help increase
understanding of this very distressing condition.

There have been suggestions that control over the bowels is what
began the civilisation of mankind, separating us from the rest of the
animal kingdom. The ability to control where and when defecation
occurred meant that early man was able to hide his faeces and their
accompanying smell from other animals, enabling him to get closer to his prey before discovery and to mask his location from the
hunters of the animal kingdom. The need to keep excreta and food
separate is also important. Getliffe & Dolman (1997) agree: 'The
importance attached to bladder and bowel control is as old as the
human race.' They cite Smith (1979) who stated: 'Incontinence is
one of the oldest medically recorded complaints in the history of
mankind.' Throughout history there have been many suggested
treatments for incontinence, particularly urinary incontinence,
from pig's urine to powdered hedgehog. The bible, too, suggests
ways of dealing with excrement! 'In the Old Testament, The Book
of Deuteronomy commands: "You must have a latrine outside the

camp and go out to this and you must have a mattock among your equipment and with this mattock when you go outside to ease yourself you must dig a hole and cover your excrement" ' (Getliffe & Dolman 1997) From this time man has continued to pursue the most efficient way of dealing with his waste matter until the development of the sophisticated flushing toilets we currently employ, first invented by Sir James Harrington in 1596 and refined by Thomas Crapper (Getliffe & Dolman 1997).

If this ability to control when and where he defecated was so important to early man, how much more vital is it considered to civilised 21st-century man with his sensitive nose? The control of bowels is considered a basic human skill over which parents worry during potty and toilet training. In many households, there are arguments over the subject, with mother and father disagreeing over methods used. Health professionals spend hours giving advice about potty training—when the child is ready and how the parents should progress with the training. However, as little, if any, time is devoted to this subject during courses in which one would expect at least basic information to be given, one might wonder how health professionals can effectively counsel parents on this. There are numerous books on the subject of potty training along with other aids to make potty training easy. Members of the family, friends and even strangers will all contribute their own views and opinions on potty training. Think also of the unwillingness of some adults to change a child's nappy when it is soiled. This therefore begins to explain why the majority of people feel such strong emotions when confronted with someone who has no bowel control at an age when it is expected they should have—that is the child who soils.

The lack of control over the escape of faeces that these children and their families face leads to a multitude of further problems. As defecation and lack of bowel control are such taboo subjects, many families feel theirs is the only child who suffers from this extremely embarrassing condition. The need to keep this secret can result in social isolation not only of the child but also of the whole family. Buchanan (1992) encapsulates the effect on the child with her statement:

For the child it is hard to imagine a social or physical problem which is more devastating to his sense of self worth and dignity than the inability to control the most basic of human functions. A child who soils lives in constant fear that he may lose control of his bowels and that at any moment he will be exposed to the fury of his parents or the taunts of his peers.

Beach (1996) tells us: 'From the child's perspective chronic constipation and soiling can be a source of constant physical and mental anguish.' Benninga et al. (1994) state:

Many doctors regard it as a trivial symptom which will eventually disappear. Apart from the shame and fear of discovery, however, it may lead to social withdrawal, low self esteem, and depression. Despite these consequences in children, encopresis and soiling have received less attention than enuresis.

Clayden (1996) also tells us:

There are few conditions which isolate children and their families more completely than constipation with overflow faecal soiling. Social contacts and even professionals may trivialise the problem and many families miss the sympathy and understanding of having to cope with such a persistent and distressing condition.

The common side-effects of constipation are a bloated feeling, nausea and lack of appetite which can mean children constantly feel unwell and never at their best. Some individuals will have other equally unpleasant side-effects (see Box 1.1). If a short spell of constipation can leave a patient feeling sluggish and out of sorts, chronic constipation can leave the sufferer feeling like this at all times. Sympathy should go to the chronic sufferer for the constant discomfort and other symptoms they endure.

Another problem faced by a number of children who soil is child abuse. A physical chastisement for failure to do what parents feel should be achieved is a real possibility. The anger generated by a child's 'accident' can quickly escalate into physical violence. Adults, if unaware of the predisposing condition which leads to the accident, can become frustrated when their child does not perform as expected. While physical abuse is one conse-

---

Box 1.1 Possible effects of constipation

Nausea	Haemorrhoids
Abdominal pain	Rectal bleeding
Reduced appetite	Urinary retention
Headache	Urinary tract infection
Bloated feeling	Urinary and/or faecal incontinence
Rectal pain	Mega rectum

quence, another possibility to be aware of, at all times, when working with children who soil, is sexual abuse. Sexual abuse can result in soiling for three reasons as Buchanan (1992) tells us:

Experience suggests there may be three possible triggers for soiling following sexual abuse. Firstly fine bowel control may be damaged by buggery; secondly the post trauma of the assault may trigger psychological mechanisms resulting in soiling; and thirdly some of the children may use soiling as a defence against unwanted sexual advances.

We obviously need to be mindful of the possibility but as professionals we have seen what happens when we do not carefully balance the possibility against the probability. High-profile cases in the past have been a sobering reminder of what can happen when only one indicator is considered and other facts are not taken into the equation. Part of the problem has been a reliance on Reflex Anal Dilatation (RAD) as an indicator of sexual abuse—it may be but it could indicate other conditions, as Illingworth (1991) reminds us:

Reflex anal dilatation was said by Hobb and Wynne to be an important indication of child sexual abuse. They described wide relaxation of the sphincter when the buttocks were gently parted, so that they could see into the rectum. They did not relate it to constipation. There has been much controversy about this. Some have found that it may be associated with severe constipation. In one study the sign was found in 16% of 129 children with severe constipation, but others found that significant constipation was less often associated with the sign. It is not always present when buggery has occurred and can occur in normal children.

In any geographical area there will be a number of children who have this distressing condition and who require a management plan to resolve the soiling problems. However, unless families strike it lucky first time or live in an area with a locally well-known 'expert' on soiling, many will see a number of different specialists. If the child has other medical conditions too, they may find the constipation and soiling almost ignored by their consultant. As the consultant is often more interested in the medical condition for which the child was initially referred, the constipation is seen as almost incidental. So many of these families are almost ready to give up asking for help with the condition by the time they finally find someone who listens. Methods of management of chronic constipation vary between practitioners. Their background influencing their choice of treatment, surgeons will treat symptoms in a different way from physicians and are perhaps more likely to resort to surgery than others. The operation used is the ACE procedure or Antegrade Colonic Enema, where a piece of bowel is brought to the surface of the abdominal wall to provide access for an enema to be given at regular intervals with the intention of emptying the bowel, commonly used for Hirschsprungs. The advantage of the ACE access is that it clears impaction from behind the blockage rather than trying to clear the faecal mass from the other side. The lack of national agreement on minimum investigations and protocols for treating the condition, except ERIC's (Enuresis Resource and Information Centre), results in 'pot-luck' healthcare received by these children and their families. However, as this area has little appeal to most professionals because, after all, they too are human, and it is not a glamorous condition, it attracts few practitioners, so finding someone with an interest in soiling can be difficult. Although chronic functional constipation with soiling is not life-threatening, it is certainly life-altering, as seen in the previous extracts. If more health professionals had a greater understanding of the condition and its effects on the child and family, perhaps these children would receive help and treatment sooner and fewer would have chronic problems. If a mother approaches a health professional for advice about an acute episode of constipation in her baby and is given effective advice, it may save months or years of involved management.

As a practitioner, showing even the slightest interest in this condition will result in an avalanche of referral letters from other professionals. Parents and children will be particularly happy to meet someone who listens and seems to know something about what is happening to them. Someone, moreover, who reassures them that the condition is curable, albeit in the long term, and offers help. One thing to be overcome is the expectation the family may have that this is a simple matter requiring a quick fix. Telling the child and parent at the outset that the treatment can take over a year is important to allay fears they may develop that their child is slow in responding. It helps to prevent their becoming disillusioned because they feel the treatment is not effective and prepares them for the long haul of the treatment.

Perhaps now is the ideal time to discuss exactly what condition we are talking about. Most children who soil suffer chronic functional constipation. Although Graham Clayden and Ulfur

Agnarsson have some very precise definitions of soiling and encopresis, in some texts and on the continent and North America the terms are often used interchangeably. Clayden & Agnarsson's definitions (1991):

Constipation. Difficulty or delay in the passage of stools (not a description of the hardness of the stool, although this is often but not always associated).

Soiling. Involuntary passage of fluid or semi-solid stool into the clothing (usually as a result of overflow from a faecally-loaded rectum).

Encopresis. Passage of a normal stool into socially inappropriate places (including clothing).

Definitions of constipation vary widely but here are a few that demonstrate the severity of the problem some of these children suffer from:

1. Iacono et al (1995) used the definition: 'one evacuation every 3–7 days—and of pain in the passage of hard stools.'
2. Loening-Baucke (1995) suggests: 'Constipation in children can be defined by a stool frequency <3 per week; but constipation also can be defined by the presence of stool retention with or without encopresis; even when stool frequency is ≥3 per week.'
3. van der Plas et al (1997) have the most descriptive definition: 'constipation was considered when children met at least two of the four following criteria: bowel frequency <3 per week; soiling and/or encopresis frequency ≥ 2 per week; large amounts of stool once per 7–30 days and an abdominal and/or rectal palpable mass. (*Clayden's definitions of soiling and encopresis apply here.*) Large amounts of stool were defined as a big lump of stool which could not easily be flushed through the toilet.'

These wide-ranging definitions also serve to illustrate the differing opinions on the condition and how to treat it. In the UK, many health professionals use Clayden's definitions as he is the acknowledged expert nationally. In other countries, there is often a similar prominent practitioner in the field whom others emulate. Different countries will also use different investigations and treatments, depending on the cultural acceptability of them.

Why is a general text on soiling needed? Approximately 3% of 5-year-olds do not have bowel control. Buchanan (1992) cites work by Bellman who 'found that bowel control seemed as a rule to be established and stabilised during the child's fourth year, and ... over 97% of boys and 99% of girls achieved bowel control by the age of seven.' As Muir & Burnett (1999), citing Sullivan, tell us, 'This problem ... is common, accounting for 3% of general paediatric referrals and up to 25% of referrals to paediatric gastroenterology centres.' Nurko (2000) suggests that 34% of English children aged 4 to 11 years have constipation and that a study of 22-month-old children found 16% were reported as being constipated. Nurko also agrees with the referral rates cited by Muir & Burnett. For health visitors and school nurses this results in a minimum of one child on their caseload. For other practitioners, including practice nurses with larger caseloads, the numbers are probably far higher and many cases go unrecognised because parents have not disclosed the fact that their child has this problem. Taubman (1997) found that 'stool toiletting refusal was surprisingly common, occurring in 106 of 428 (22%) children. However; in only 29 of these children did the parents consult their paediatricians for advice.'

The need to be able either to manage the case or, at the very least, to understand the reason behind another's treatment so that support can be given to these children and their families is important. By supporting what the practitioner managing the child's condition has said with regard to the treatment, another health professional is playing a major role in the plan. Even brief interventions can contribute to successful treatment. It is accepted that this is not an area that attracts every practitioner but if you have contact with families undergoing a management programme they need your encouragement to continue. For this, a basic knowledge of the condition and management techniques is required. Early support and advice for the mother of a baby showing signs of constipation can be vital.

While some children have suffered for relatively short periods of time e.g. under a year, there are many more who have suffered for a number of years. Seeking help, perhaps after numerous failed attempts, can be daunting for both the children and their families as the fear of rejection and failure is ever present. Children attending one clinic have ranged from 4-year-olds with a problem since birth to 12-year-olds with constipation since the age of four years. These differences clearly illustrate the lack of local services prior to a special clinic being set up. Although some community paediatricians are interested, their general clinic waiting list is often too long to allow frequent follow-up appointments for children with soiling problems. Regular follow-up is vital in the successful treatment of chronic functional constipation with soiling. Bear in mind what happens if you are told to do something before your next out-patient appointment—perhaps you are to lose weight or try a new diet—if the next appointment is in 6 months, how long are you tempted to put it off before you start? Others are no different to you. As already stated, the commonest cause of soiling is constipation with faecal impaction leading to overflow as Buchanan (1992) explains: 'the basic problem is one of constipation which becomes so severe as to lead to a partial blockage of the bowel. As a result of the blockage some of the motions liquefy and seep past to produce faecal soiling.' Constipation over long periods, whether primarily caused by poor diet and fluid intake, a slow transit time or by another organic condition, will result in the rectum enlarging to the extent that it may be described as a mega rectum. Treatment programmes are aimed at reversing the enlargement to normal functional capacity.

Diet plays an important role in bowel health and in avoiding constipation and, for the enlightened, fibre forms a large enough proportion of their dietary intake to maintain regular bowel evacuations. However, many families do not have sufficient knowledge or the resources to maintain adequate fibre intake within a balanced diet. Fluid intake, too, can be problematic—a colleague with a longstanding problem of constipation had a poor fluid intake because 'I don't have time to keep skipping off to the ladies'. 'To try to rectify these inadequacies, a high proportion of health professionals' time can be spent in health promotion on dietary issues. This is particularly the case when there is a familial problem of constipation and in those children with slow transit time, i.e. when their food progresses more slowly than the 'average' person's along the intestinal tract. This can result in the stool becoming very hard as there is a longer time for water reabsorption. The diet needs careful adjustments in these cases—see Chapter 6.

A rarer cause of constipation leading to soiling and in the longer term mega rectum is Hirschsprung's disease. In this condition there is an absence of neural ganglions in sections of the colon and rectum. It can affect varying lengths of the large intestine from a large proportion to very small sections—ultra short segment Hirschsprung's. This can only be correctly diagnosed by biopsy and is usually diagnosed in the very young (following an episode of severe acute constipation). The clinical picture in soiling can, however, give rise to the suspicion of short or ultra short segment Hirschsprung's disease.

NORMAL DEVELOPMENT OF BOWEL CONTROL

All babies start with a reflex arc within bowel control; that is, when the rectum senses the presence of a faecal mass within it, the message is passed via the parasympathetic nerve pathway to the brain and the return message allows defecation to occur. This is often stimulated by feeding so that after the baby has had a feed, the gastrocolic reflex moves intestinal contents along the colon to the rectum. This situation is somewhat ironic when one considers that many parents will change babies' nappies prior to feeding them. This situation will last through the first year of life.

As they develop during their second year, babies learn to recognise the presence of a faecal mass in the rectum and, while the passage of stools is still almost a reflex, they are seen to have some knowledge that it is happening. The next year of life sees the development of the ability to hold on to the faecal mass for long periods until they feel they are ready to release it. The concept of social acceptability has now started to develop. Finally, during the fourth year of life, they learn to hold on and to release the faeces when they desire.

COMMON TIMES OF ONSET OF CONSTIPATION

As a health professional it is useful to realise that there are certain times in a child's life when constipation is more likely to develop. When one looks at the child's life pattern, the times are fairly predictable and therefore these should be the times when health promotion messages about diet or fluid are particularly concentrated:

1. Constipation from birth must be taken seriously as it may be a symptom of Hirschsprung's disease which, in severe cases, can lead to intestinal obstruction and death. In fact, a delay in passing meconium for over 48 hours after birth should be noted and the information conveyed to the consultant paediatrician or general practitioner.

2. At 2 weeks when the child is at home and perhaps the mother's partner has returned to work and she is alone. There may be a switch from exclusive breastfeeding. The child may develop a feverish illness which, unless the mother is vigilant in increasing the fluid intake to compensate for the fluid lost by the raised temperature, can result in an acute period of constipation.

3. At 2 months when many mothers stop breastfeeding and introduce formula milk: 'The stools of the fully breastfed baby remain loose but change in character immediately after other foods are given. Even a small amount of cows' milk makes them firmer' (Illingworth 1991).

4. At 4 months when the baby is beginning to be weaned and foods other than milk become part of his diet. If the mother is not careful this too can lead to constipation, particularly if other fluids are not introduced into the child's diet at the same time.

5. At 2 years of age when toilet training starts. This can become a time when the child wilfully withholds stools, leading to harder stools which are painful to pass and so he withholds again. This can become a vicious circle which needs careful management. Other physical causes including anal fistula or fissure and streptococcal infections of the skin around the anus may also lead to stool withholding.

It can be seen that many factors can contribute to the child's condition. It could be diet, drinking, abuse, organic causes or psychological aspects. Perhaps each one has a part to play and therefore health professionals need to be aware of these factors and to ensure that the management programmes instituted help to alleviate them. The following chapters will examine different aspects of the condition and its management.

CONCLUSION

While bowel control is a basic human skill that most children have learned by the age of 5 years, some have not. Throughout history there have been attempts to aid control of the bladder and bowels. The commonest cause of soiling in children is constipation with faecal loading, leading to overflow. There are many factors in the onset of the child's problem and many children have suffered for a number of years. The child has normally seen a number of different practitioners before encountering someone with knowledge of the subject and therefore lots of support and understanding is needed.

REFERENCES

Beach R C 1996 Management of Childhood Constipation. The Lancet 348(9030): 766–767
Benninga M A, Buller H A, Heymens H S A, Tytgat G N J, Taminiau J A J M 1994 Is encopresis always the result of constipation? Archives of Disease in Childhood 71(2): 186–193
Buchanan A 1992 Children who Soil, Assessment and Treatment. John Wiley, Chichester
Clayden G, Agnarsson U 1991 Constipation in Childhood. Oxford University Press, Oxford
Clayden G 1996 A guide for good practice: childhood constipation. Ambulatory Child Health 1(5): 250–255
ERIC 2001 Childhood soiling, minimum standards of practice for treatment and service delivery: benchmarking guidelines. ERIC (Enuresis Resource and Information Centre), 34 Old School House, Britannia Road, Kingswood, Bristol BS15 8DB, UK. Tel. 0117 960 3060, fax. 0117 960 0401, email info@eric.org.uk, www.eric.org.uk
Getliffe K, Dolman M 1997 Promoting continence: a clinical and research resource. Baillière Tindall, London
Iacono G, Carroccio A, Cavataio F, Montalto G, Cantarero M D, Notarbartolo A 1995 Chronic constipation as a symptom of cow milk allergy. The Journal of Pediatrics 126(1): 34–39
Illingworth R 1991 The Normal Child (some problems of the early years and their treatment), 10 edn. Churchill Livingstone, Edinburgh
Loening-Baucke V 1995 Biofeedback treatment for chronic constipation and encopresis in childhood: long-term outcome. Pediatrics 96(1): 105–110
Kamm M A, Lennard-Jones J E (eds) 1994 Constipation. Wrightson Biomedical Publishing, Petersfield
Muir J, Burnett C 1999 Setting up a nurse-led clinic for intractable childhood constipation. British Journal of Community Nursing 4(8): 395–399
Nurko S 2000 Current Gastroenterology Reports 2: 234–240
Smith P S 1979 The development of urinary incontinence in the mentally ill. Unpublished PhD thesis, University of Newcastle
Taubman B 1997 Toilet training and toiletting refusal for stool only: a prospective study. Pediatrics 99(1): 54–58
van der Plas R N, Benninga M A, Redekop W K, Taminiau J A, Buller H A 1997 How accurate is the recall of bowel habits in children with defaecation disorders? European Journal of Paediatrics 156: 178–181

2

Anatomy and physiology

The structure of the colon	Defecation
The role of the pelvic floor	Patterns of defecation
muscles	Constipation
Efficacy of the gastrointestinal	Hirschsprung's disease
tract	

In order to ensure that there is complete understanding of the condition discussed in this text, a thorough understanding of the gastrointestinal tract is vital. So that this can be achieved, this chapter will give the factual knowledge required to understand the condition fully. Many practitioners will have trained a number of years ago and therefore require a refresher, but it is surprising how quickly it comes back when one is reminded of the subject. Some practitioners may not feel the need to refresh their knowledge but the information is here if required.

While the whole of the gastrointestinal tract is involved in the digestion of food, much of the first part of the tract can be studied briefly so that the colon and rectum may be considered in more detail later as these are the more relevant components in this condition.

The component parts of the gastrointestinal tract are the mouth, pharynx, oesophagus, stomach, small intestine, large intestine, rectum and anal canal (see Fig. 2.1). The mouth starts off the process of digestion and the 'processing' of food to faeces, by mastication and the action of the enzymes contained in the saliva, which is produced in glands emptying into the buccal cavity. Once it has been chewed, the food is swallowed and passes through the pharynx down the oesophagus to the stomach where the food is churned to ensure all the surface area is in contact with more enzymes and the hydrochloric acid produced to continue the process. This phase of food entering the stomach and the actions which follow can result in the gastrocolic reflex that leads to the desire to defecate in some instances. The contents of the stomach at this time are called

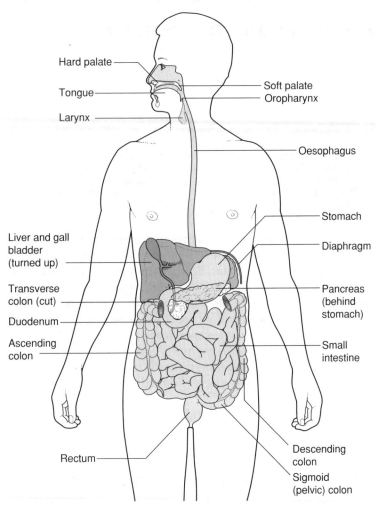

Figure 2.1 The organs of the digestive system. (From Wilson & Waugh 1996, Churchill Livingstone.)

chyme. A few substances, including water, alcohol and some lipid-soluble drugs are absorbed from the stomach. Meals remain in the stomach for varying times, depending on the main component of the food. Fatty meals remain longest, a meal with protein will leave in a shorter time and the quickest to empty from the stomach will be a carbohydrate-based meal, which will empty in 2–3 hours.

Box 2.1 Points to remember

- Component parts of the gastrointestinal tract are: the mouth, pharynx, oesophagus, stomach, small intestine, large intestine, rectum and anal canal
- Digestion begins in the mouth
- Food passes via the pharynx and oesophagus to the stomach
- Food stays in the stomach for varying lengths of time depending on its constituents: fatty meals remain the longest and carbohydrate the shortest
- The entry of food into the stomach triggers the gastrocolic reflex
- Some absorption takes place from the stomach, mainly water, alcohol and lipid-soluble drugs

---

The small intestine continues from the stomach at the pyloric sphincter and leads to the large intestine at the ileocaecal valve, which controls the speed of emptying of contents from the ileum to the colon. The small intestine is a little over 5 m long and it lies in folds within the abdominal cavity. It is divided into three parts which are continuous. The first is the duodenum which is approximately 25 cm long. This is the section into which both bile and pancreatic secretions are emptied via the common bile and pancreatic ducts. The jejunum is the next section and this is approximately 2 m long. This leads into the ileum which is 3 m long. While the chyme is in the small intestine, chemical digestion continues and most nutrient absorption occurs.

The large intestine then arises in the right iliac fossa at the ileocaecal valve which also acts to prevent back flow from the large to small intestine. The colon then ascends to the hepatic flexure in the right upper quadrant of the abdomen; this section is called the ascending colon. The transverse colon crosses to the left upper quadrant towards the spleen where the splenic flexure is found before it descends (the descending colon) to the left iliac fossa. As it enters the pelvis it becomes the sigmoid colon and turns

---

Box 2.2 Points to remember

- The small intestine is a little over 5 m long
- It comprises the duodenum (25 cm long), the jejunum (2 m long) and the ileum (3 m long)
- Digestion continues and most absorption occurs while chyme is in the small intestine
- Bile and pancreatic secretions are added to the chyme while it is in the small intestine

---

towards the midline to form an 'S' shape which is vital in maintaining continence, and becomes the rectum and anal canal. This is 1.5 m in length in total with a lumen larger than the small intestine at approximately 6 cm diameter (see Fig. 2.2).

The rectum is approximately 13 cm long and the lumen is dilated in relation to the rest of the colon. The anal canal leads from the rectum to the exterior of the body and is only approximately 4 cm long. The anus is under the control of two sphincters; the internal one is under autonomic control while the external one is under voluntary control (see Fig. 2.3). Besides transporting the

---

Box 2.3 Points to remember

- The large intestine comprises the ascending, transverse, descending and sigmoid colon, the rectum and anal canal
- The colon measures approximately 1.5 m in length and is approximately 6 cm in diameter
- It arises in the right iliac fossa at the ileocaecal valve which prevents backflow
- The main function is transport although some absorption takes place

---

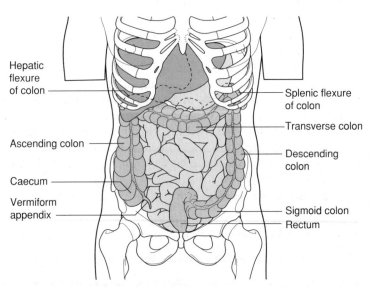

Figure 2.2 The parts of the large intestine (colon) and their positions. (From Wilson & Waugh 1996, Churchill Livingstone.)

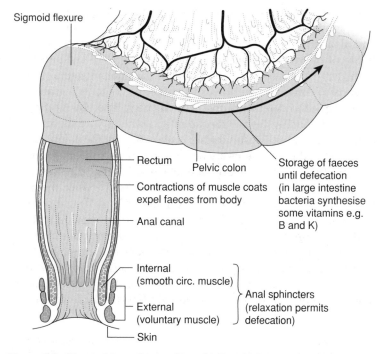

Sigmoid flexure

Rectum

Pelvic colon

Contractions of muscle coats
expel faeces from body

Anal canal

Internal
(smooth circ. muscle)

External
(voluntary muscle)

Skin

Storage of faeces
until defecation
(in large intestine
bacteria synthesise
some vitamins e.g.
B and K)

Anal sphincters
(relaxation permits
defecation)

Figure 2.3 The rectum and anus. (From McNaught & Callander 1975, Churchill Livingstone.)

faeces out of the body, the other function of the large intestine is absorption of water, mineral salts, vitamins and some drugs.

THE STRUCTURE OF THE COLON

The colon has four layers; the peritoneum is the outer layer providing a cover for many of the abdominal cavity's contents. Below this is the muscle layer. The muscle layer has, in fact, two layers of fibres: the longitudinal fibres form the outer layer and the circular fibres form the inner layer. These muscle fibres are smooth muscles and are therefore under involuntary control. The next layer is the submucous layer formed of connective tissue and some elastic fibres. This layer contains the nerve plexuses and the blood supply as well as lymph vessels and lymphoid tissue. The nerves are both sympathetic and parasympathetic. The inner lining is the mucosa which in the large intestine lacks villi.

The arrangement of the two types of muscle fibres ensures that mass movement can be present to move the colon contents along and also to make the contents come into contact with the mucosa lining of the colon to help absorption (see Fig. 2.4). The peristalsis in the large intestine differs from that in the small intestine because it tends to come in long waves to move the contents towards the rectum prior to defecation and is often precipitated by food entering the stomach—the gastrocolic reflex. Only 4% of the material entering the gastrointestinal tract is absorbed by the colon. It is in the colon that the contents are acted upon by bacteria and some of the products of this action are absorbed here, e.g. vitamins. Bacterial gut flora acting upon the chyme also produce the gases that form flatus at a rate of approximately 400 to 700 ml per day. The gases are composed of nitrogen and carbon dioxide together with small amounts of more flammable gases including methane, hydrogen and hydrogen sulphide. Some foods will result in higher quantities of gaseous production, particularly foods with high levels of carbohydrates which are metabolised to polysaccharides and eventually saccharides. The polysaccharides are fermented by

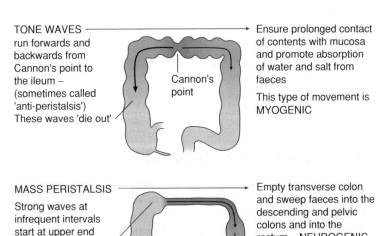

TONE WAVES run forwards and backwards from Cannon's point to the ileum – (sometimes called 'anti-peristalsis') These waves 'die out'

Cannon's point

→ Ensure prolonged contact of contents with mucosa and promote absorption of water and salt from faeces

This type of movement is MYOGENIC

MASS PERISTALSIS

Strong waves at infrequent intervals start at upper end of ascending colon

→ Empty transverse colon and sweep faeces into the descending and pelvic colons and into the rectum – NEUROGENIC

[reflex often initiated by passage of food into stomach (gastrocolic reflex)]

Figure 2.4   Mass waves. (From McNaught & Callander 1975, Churchill Livingstone.)

Box 2.4 Points to remember

- There are four layers in the structure of the colon: the outer layer is the peritoneum, the next layer has muscle fibres in two directions, circular and longitudinal, the next carries the nerve plexuses, both sympathetic and parasympathetic, and the blood and lymph vessels, the innermost layer is the mucous membrane
- Movement of contents is by both mass movement and tone waves
- Only 4% of the contents entering the colon are absorbed
- Bacteria act upon the contents and create flatus at a rate of approximately 400–700 ml. Carbohydrates produce most gas

---

the bacteria to cause the gas production. Baked beans are renowned for having this effect on someone who has eaten them, with good reason as they contain so much unrefined carbohydrate.

THE ROLE OF THE PELVIC FLOOR MUSCLES

The muscles of the pelvic floor play a vital role in maintaining continence. They not only support the organs of the pelvis within the abdominal cavity but we know they form part of the sphincter control in the bladder. The anal canal passes through the levator ani muscle, the major muscle of the pelvic floor. One part of the levator ani, the puborectalis, starts at the pubic bone and forms a loop around the rectum at its junction with the anus and back to the pubic bone to maintain the 'S' shape mentioned earlier. This prevents the loss of faecal matter by keeping the anorectal angle acute enough to ensure the internal anal sphincter is closed (see Fig. 2.5). Getliffe & Dolman (1997) state that:

This thick band of muscle is responsible for creating an angle; ranging from approximately 60 to 110 degrees between the rectum and the upper anal canal. This angle is known as the 'anorectal' angle and is formed as a result of the rectum being pulled toward the pubic bone. As long as the angle remains below 110 degrees, faeces from the rectum cannot pass into the anal canal; and this is achieved by contraction of the puborectalis muscle.

If the call to pass stool is ignored and faecal matter has already started the descent to the anal canal, it can be seen that this will keep the anorectal angle at more than 110 degrees and the seepage of material past it is easily achieved. If the pelvic floor muscles are lax it can also be envisaged that the angle required to maintain faecal continence may not be present.

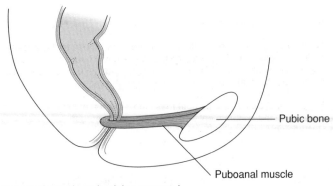

Puboanal muscle maintaining anorectal
angle; note 'S' shape to colon and rectum

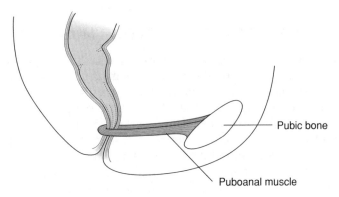

Lax puboanal muscle failing to maintain anorectal angle

Figure 2.5   The role of the puboanal muscle in maintaining faecal
continence.

Box 2.5   Points to remember

- The major muscle of the pelvic floor is the levator ani, part of which, the
  pubo rectalis, starts on the inner surface of the pubic bone and travels
  back forming a loop around the rectum and ends on the inner surface of
  the pubic bone again
- This maintains the anorectal angle at between 60 to 110°, keeping the
  contents of the sigmoid colon there and not allowing seepage
- If this angle is not maintained because of constipation or a lax pelvic floor
  then continence may be lost

EFFICACY OF THE GASTROINTESTINAL TRACT

The average adult consumes approximately 1.2 L water and 0.8 L food each day. To this are added various secretions from the gastrointestinal tract and other organs which play a role in the digestion of food as follows: 1.5 L saliva, 2 L gastric secretions, 0.5 L bile, 1.5 L pancreatic secretions and 1.5 L intestinal secretions. This makes a grand total of 9 L of food and fluid put into the gastrointestinal tract. However, since faeces are composed of only 0.1 L water and 50 g solids, the remainder must be reabsorbed and so it is: 8.5 L in the small intestine and, from the 0.5 L entering it, 350 mL in the large intestine.

The solids in faeces are composed of fibre, microbes (both dead and alive), epithelial cells, fatty acids and mucus secreted by the intestine to lubricate the passage through the colon, with 60 to 70% of the composition of faeces being water, despite the reabsorption already described. The brown colour comes from stercobilin.

DEFECATION

When the stomach empties, the segmentation movements of the ileum increases; this is known as the gastroileal reflex. This reflex is under the influence of gastrin, a secretion of the stomach, but it can also be affected by emotions. The increased motility of the small intestine leads to the ileocaecal valve opening and chyme entering the colon.

Most of the time the rectum is empty, however at intervals a mass movement, which is a wave of intense contraction of the smooth muscles, pushes a volume of the sigmoid colon's contents into the rectum. The reflex happens at the same time as the

---

Box 2.6 Points to remember

- The gastrointestinal tract is very efficient at reabsorbing almost all the fluid that enters it
- As well as water within the food we eat, fluids that are mixed with it include: saliva, gastric secretions, bile, pancreatic secretions and intestinal secretions adding up to approximately 9 L of fluid
- Only 100 mL of water is contained in faeces
- Faeces is composed of epithelial cells, bacteria, mucus, fatty acids, undigested food and stercobilin, which gives the brown colour

gastroileal reflex. The movement differs from a peristaltic wave because the smooth muscle remains contracted for a while after the movement is completed, unlike peristalsis where the muscle relaxes as soon as the contraction wave has passed (see Fig. 2.4). All of this indicates that the movements are much slower than the contractions of the small intestine and, in fact, the contents may stay in the large intestine for up to 18 to 24 hours, providing time for the gut flora to act on the contents and multiply.

As the bolus of the contents enters the rectum, pressure receptors sense the presence of something in the rectum. The internal sphincter relaxes while the external sphincter contracts, allowing approximately 30 mL of the contents to pass over special sensitive nerve endings which can distinguish whether the contents are gaseous (flatus), liquid (diarrhoea) or solid (faeces). This process is usually referred to as 'sampling' and is carried out subconsciously. The internal anal sphincter then contracts again until the act of defecation occurs. The mass movement of faeces into the rectum stimulates the conscious urge to defecate by stretched mechanoreceptors in the walls activated by the distension that occurs. Vander et al (1990) describe the defecation reflex as follows:

The reflex response consists of a contraction of the rectum, relaxation of the internal anal sphincter, contraction of the external anal sphincter, and increased peristaltic activity in the sigmoid colon. Eventually a pressure is reached in the rectum that triggers relaxation of the external anal sphincter, however, allowing the faeces to be expelled.

The conscious urge to defecate can be delayed by messages from brain centres to somatic nerves which override the afferent nerve impulses of the defecation reflex. This keeps the external anal sphincter closed until such time as the individual reaches a socially acceptable place to allow the reflex to be completed. If the urge is resisted long enough then the rectum walls will relax and the need to defecate passes until such time as another mass movement occurs, emptying further faeces into the rectum.

The process of defecation is complex and occurs when an individual finds a convenient time and location in which to allow themselves to sit comfortably for the effort required. The contracting of the internal anal sphincter results in a raised pressure within the rectum (see Fig. 2.6). This leads to an increase in both sensation and the intensity of the muscular action and the urge to

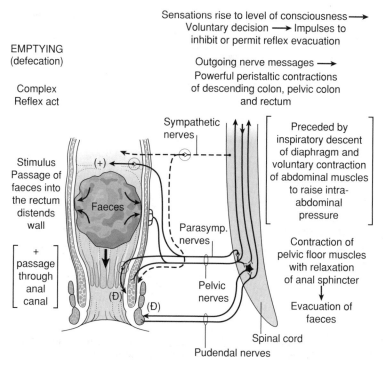

Figure 2.6 The process of defecation. (From McNaught & Callander 1975, Churchill Livingstone.)

defecate becomes stronger. Rectal pressure is now higher than the anal pressure and, aided by Valsalva manoeuvre, the faeces will be expelled. Valsalva's manoeuvre involves the glottis being closed following a deep inspiration and the abdominal and thoracic muscles being contracted, leading to raised intraabdominal and intrathoracic pressure, exerting pressure and movement on the faecal mass towards the anal canal. At this time the puborectalis muscle relaxes, increasing the anorectal angle and allowing the pelvic floor to descend to ease the process. The faeces are expelled and the external anal sphincter contracts, the internal anal sphincter begins to close and the rectum returns to its empty state.

Position is vital when one is preparing to defecate. Both Chiarelli & Markwell (1992) and Getliffe & Dolman (1997) state that the squatting position (see Fig. 2.7) is the most effective in

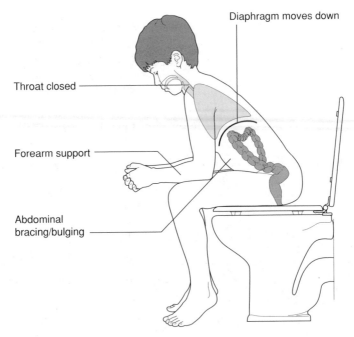

Diaphragm moves down

Throat closed

Forearm support

Abdominal bracing/bulging

Figure 2.7 The right way to open the bowels. (From Getliffe & Dolman 1997, Baillière Tindall, with permission of Chiarelli & Markwell 1992.)

aiding defecation as 'it allows the anal canal to be opened more fully from front to back, making a much more efficient funnel' (Chiarelli & Markwell 1992). When working with children, it is important that this information is shared with parents. It should also be recommended that something be provided to stand on when squatting. If the individual feels the need to defecate at a time that is not convenient then these sensations may have to be suppressed. While it is not recommended that ignoring the need to defecate is something that should frequently be done, there will be times when it is essential that the individual ignores the 'call to stool'. If the individual has to inhibit the reflexes described so far for long periods of time, there develops fatigue of the external anal sphincter. Clayden & Agnarsson (1991) tell us, 'However, the external sphincter does fatigue when maximally contracted, after about 50 seconds in adults and about 30 seconds in children.' Their physiology means the anal canal and rectum are well able to cope with this. The external anal sphincter, which is normally

---

Box 2.7   Points to remember

- Defecation occurs after contents of colon are moved into the rectum, usually following gastrocolic reflex
- The rectum, which is normally closed and empty, senses the presence of faeces via mechanoreceptors in its walls
- 'Sampling' occurs subconsciously to detect if the substance present is gas, liquid or solid
- Following this the internal anal sphincter contracts again and rectal pressure rises: this results in relaxation of the internal anal sphincter and an increase in the peristaltic movement of the faeces into the anal canal and strong urges to defecate
- Valsalva's manoeuvre aids expulsion of the faeces when a convenient time and place is reached
- The pubo rectalis relaxes at this time to allow a greater angle and the passage of the faecal mass through the anorectal angle
- Position is vital to aid defecation—squatting with the forearms braced upon the thighs and the heels raised from the floor

---

relaxed during defecation, contracts resulting in a raised anal pressure but a lower rectal pressure. The puborectalis contracts which leads to a reduced anorectal angle as the rectum is pulled towards the public bone. This, together with some reverse peristalsis, moves the faeces back to the sigmoid colon, although some may remain in the rectum too.

Patterns of defecation

Throughout life the number and frequency of bowel evacuations will change as a natural developmental process. The neonate's first bowel evacuation is the meconium plug which is a grey-white or yellow substance, followed by meconium, a dark green-black substance which is sticky but almost non odorous. The majority of newborn babies will have opened their bowels within the first 24 hours. Illingworth (1991) states: 'The majority of babies pass the first stool during the first day of life; 69% of 500 full term babies passed the first stool in 12 hours, and 94% within 24 hours of birth.' If there is a delay in having the bowels opened for more than 48 hours after birth, Hirschsprung's disease should be considered and excluded. The stool will gradually change in appearance over the next days and up to 3 weeks, through less intense green-black to green-brown, to the normal yellow colour expected of a baby's stool. If the child is fully breastfed, the stool will also remain soft. To begin with, all babies

---

Box 2.8 Points to remember

- All individuals have different patterns of defecation
- The first stool is the meconium plug, then meconium followed by a typical baby's yellow stool approximately 4 times a day. This changes as the child grows until their normal pattern is reached at approximately 3 or 4 years of age
- Delay in the passing of meconium should be investigated. 94% of neonates have opened their bowels within 24 hours of birth

---

have frequent explosive bowel evacuations. Different foodstuffs or medications may change the colour of the stool and parents, as well as professionals, should be made aware of this. As a more varied diet is introduced at weaning so the stool will change again, eventually becoming the colour and consistency expected of faeces: a brown, formed stool of varying hardness, passed anything between 3 times a day to 3 times a week (see Table 2.1).

CONSTIPATION

As discussed in the previous chapter, constipation should be considered as the delay in the passage of stool, not as the degree of hardness, although the two are often associated. Delay in the passage of stool results in the faeces staying longer in the colon, with more water being absorbed all the time it is there, despite the large intestine not being very efficient at reabsorption. As more water is removed from the faecal mass, it becomes harder and more painful to pass. If pain has been experienced previously at defecation (possibly caused by a fissure or an acute infection of the anus with streptococcus), it is easy to see that the child may become wary of passing another and of suffering the same discomfort. So constipation leads to constipation. There is a mistaken belief by the public that everyone must have their bowels opened once every day and if it does not happen they reach for

Table 2.1 Changing patterns of stools passed per day

Age	Number of stools (normal range)
First few weeks of life	4 stools per day
4 months	2 stools per day
4 years	1 stool per day
3–4 years	3 stools per day to 3 stools per week

the medicine to make it happen. As illustrated in Table 2.1, the normal range of frequency of bowel evacuations varies between individuals from 2 or 3 times daily to only 3 times a week. A temporary change in the normal regularity of bowel evacuations should be considered for minor investigative work and treatment as necessary but chronic changes must be fully investigated. There are many and varied causes for an acute episode of constipation as illustrated in Table 2.2.

Clayden & Agnarsson (1991) suggest that there may be a normal distribution curve of rectal size which would be impossible to prove due to ethical reasons but this would certainly help to explain why there is some familial tendency towards constipation. Those with the congenitally larger rectal capacity would require a larger faecal mass to stimulate the urge to defecate and to inhibit the internal anal sphincter. The other possibility is that in response to a single or repeated large faecal mass, because of acute or chronic constipation, the rectum stretches to accommodate the mass and

Table 2.2 Possible causes of constipation in children

Type of problem	Specific causes
Emotional	Depression, behavioural aspects
Ignoring sensations	Previous painful defecation e.g. hard stool, fistula, fissure, streptococcal infection of the skin around the anus
Diet	Poor dietary intake of fibre, fussy eaters. Travel.
Hormonal problems	Hypothyroidism, hyperparathyroidism, Addison's disease, diabetes mellitus
Gut motility	Child inactive, insufficient exercise taken to aid motility
Medication	Analgesics, antacids, antidepressants, antimuscarinic drugs, antihypertensives (although not many children will be taking these), anxiolytics, sedatives and neuroleptics, diuretics and iron supplements
The environmental factors	School toilets! Toilet not available or suitable for child to perform in comfort. Travel
Postoperative	Following surgery of any type that has interfered with the bowel
Bowel disorders	Irritable bowel syndrome, mega colon, mega rectum, slow and normal time constipation, fistulas and fissures
Neuropathic problems	Congenital or acquired spinal accidents

thereafter requires a larger mass to stimulate it. Defecation therefore becomes an infrequent event for the child.

Although children with chronic constipation do respond well to therapeutic interventions aimed at stimulating a response to smaller faecal masses, and this would support the hypothesis that the rectum enlarges as a direct result of constipation, relapses years later support the larger than average rectal capacity theory. Clayden & Agnarsson (1991) suggest that 'The truth probably lies somewhere between these two views, with each child having a degree of both congenital and acquired causes of the large capacity.'

Hirschsprung's disease

A simple explanation of this condition is that it is the absence of neural ganglions in the colon; however, the length of the segment affected may vary and its effects are therefore variable. It affects approximately 1 in 5000 live births, although more boys than girls are affected; it is associated with Down's syndrome and is usually diagnosed soon after birth. In later childhood, short segment or ultra-short segment Hirschsprung's disease may be suspected from the clinical picture presented on assessment; specific tests will confirm it.

The nerve supply to the bowel, as we have described earlier, lies in the second layer in from the interior lumen of the intestine. As the fetus is developing, the parasympathetic nerve plexuses start growing from the craniocervical area and spread downwards as the bowel develops, being fully formed and innervating the whole bowel at approximately 12 weeks gestation. It can be seen, then, that if the nerve development does not match the bowel development a variable length of bowel may be affected. Muscle without nerve supply tends to contract, so the area of

---

Box 2.9 Points to remember

- Constipation is the delay in passing a stool and, although often associated with it, does not refer to the hardness of the stool
- Constipation can lead to more constipation
- There are many causes of constipation
- Constipation can be both acute and chronic
- Changes in normal bowel habits should be investigated
- It is uncertain whether constipation leads to a larger capacity rectum or if the larger capacity was present and led to the constipation

aganglionic bowel will be narrowed, while the area with a good supply of nerve fibres will appear to be dilated in comparison. If the nerve impulses are stopped at a point in the bowel and peristalsis or mass movements cannot move the contents all the way to the rectum and anus, it can be easily imagined that a blockage will result. There will, at the point of the colon without parasympathetic nerve supply, form a large blockage of faecal matter which cannot pass through the narrow segment. As the nerve fibres are very close beneath the mucosa, a biopsy is a relatively easy task for a skilled paediatric surgeon and the absence of the parasympathetic nerve fibres can be demonstrated by an experienced pathologist.

Clayden & Agnarsson (1991) tell us that the longer the segment affected by Hirschsprung's disease, the earlier a diagnosis is usually made but the symptoms, whatever the length of the affected segment, may include any of the following:

- delay in passing meconium
- constipation starting within the first week of life
- vomiting (a good indication of intestinal obstruction)
- alternating constipation and diarrhoea
- severe abdominal distension
- weight gain not following centiles
- a temporary improvement after rectal examination (often followed by an explosive passage of liquid faeces and gas)
- less faecal overflow soiling than expected with the degree of faecal loading (in older children).

Box 2.10 Points to remember

- Hirschsprung's disease affects 1 in 5000 live births. Short segment affects more boys than girls but long segment affects boys and girls in equal ratio
- This condition results from an absence of parasympathetic nerve ganglions
- The area with no nerve supply will be constricted and narrow
- There will be a large faecal mass and mega rectum/colon behind the constriction
- Long segment Hirschsprung's will present earlier than short segment and can become a medical emergency as the bowel becomes obstructed
- Diagnosis is made by specific tests or rectal biopsy

The shorter the segment affected, the more difficulty there may be in differentiating the symptoms, which are more subtle, from those of other conditions.

REFERENCES

Chiarelli P, Markwell S 1992 Let's get things moving: overcoming constipation. Gore & Osment Publications, Woollahra, NSW
Clayden G, Agnarsson U 1991 Constipation in childhood. Oxford University Press, Oxford
Getliffe K, Dolman M 1997 Promoting continence: a clinical and research resource. Baillière Tindall, London
Illingworth R 1991 The normal child (some problems of the early years and their treatment), 10th edn. Churchill Livingstone, Edinburgh
McNaught A B, Callander R 1975 Nurses' illustrated physiology, 3rd edn. Churchill Livingstone, Edinburgh
Vander A J, Sherman J H, Luciano D S 1990 Human physiology: the mechanisms of body function 5th edn. McGraw-Hill Publishing, New York
Wilson K J W, Waugh A 1996 Ross & Wilson Anatomy and physiology in health and illness, 8th edn. Churchill Livingstone, Edinburgh

3

Assessment

INTRODUCTION

The first stage of successful management of the child with chronic functional constipation with overflow soiling starts with an extensive and thorough assessment. Many of the children who present with this condition, as already stated, have had the problem for a number of years. Both the child and parents or carers can reach the stage of feeling that this problem is one for which there is no treatment and one which will always be present. A full explanation, therefore, is imperative, as well as the warning that there is no magic solution and the management will take over a year in most cases. Explaining at the outset what the treatment regime may entail is vital to prepare both child and parent for what can be a long and difficult episode. For many families, finding someone who is interested in soiling and enthusiastic about its treatment will be the beginning of treatment for them and will start helping to raise their self-esteem. Many families who have sought help in the past have found that no-one appears to have taken more than a passing interest in a problem that dominates their lives. Most parents are more than willing to discuss in great detail the history of their child's condition. The art of assessment is to direct the conversation to useful facts—yes, if great aunt Freda also had a problem, that indicates there is a familial trend towards constipation. However, it does not help to hear who treated her and what treatment she had as different treatment regimes are now used and there is wide variation between adult and children's constipation treatments. The use of good visual aids for this explanation of the condition and treatment helps to reinforce the message.

PREPARATION

For an inexperienced practitioner, a detailed assessment will take at least 1 hour but with increased proficiency comes increased speed. An assessment tool that allows you to follow the same format at each assessment helps to ensure the collection of the required information (see Fig. 3.1A–D). If none is available locally then a new one could be designed. If it is well designed it can be used for all continence problems in children.

FIRST INTERVIEW OR APPOINTMENT

With sufficient time set aside and the appropriate assessment form prepared, the interview can commence. Basic demographic information, if available, can be collected prior to the interview, but be aware of the population you serve: are they mobile, frequently moving house or do they remain at the same address for many years? If these details were obtained prior to the appointment there may have been a change of address.

It is useful to discover who else lives at home and any relevant family history. Often parents have a tendency to constipation although possibly not to the same degree as their offspring. Siblings may also not have as regular bowel movements as the average child. Assessment forms (see Fig. 3.1A–D) should include sections to record any bedtime routines specific to the child so that all continence problems are covered, including nocturnal enuresis. Asking the parent what they feel the problem is can be very revealing. Although most seem very supportive of the child with overflow soiling, some degree of parental intolerance may be discovered, indicated by their perception of the condition being a nuisance to themselves, not as a real life-changing problem for the child.

The child's view may also be revealing, but it is important to remember that many children adopt an air of unconcern as a defence mechanism, to hide their true feelings of despair that

Childrens Continence Assessment Form

Computer Number ....

Name ....

Date .... DoB................ Sex ....

Address ....

....

Telephone ....

School ....

....

GP .... HV .... SN ....

Surgery ....

....

....

Other Agencies ....

....

....

Referred by ....

Family Members ....

....

Age First Seen ....

Relevant Family History ....

....

	Yes	No	
Shared Bedroom	☐	☐	Stressful Events ....
Shared bed	☐	☐	....
Laundry Facilities	☐	☐	Bedroom Routine ....
Waste Collection	☐	☐	....
Storage Facilities	☐	☐	....

Toilet Facilities eg, indoor/outdoor, shared, access, potty, supports

....

....

Other relevant family circumstances ie, problems at school, changes expected

....

....

Other Comments eg, toilet rituals

....

....

....

....

....

....

Parent/Carer view of condition

....

....

Child's view ....

....

....

School's view ....

....

Medical History and General Health	Current Medications (including over-the-counter and herbal)
....	....
....	....
....	....
Fluid intake - amount, type and when	**Development Milestones, including current levels of:** mobility, dexterity and communication
....	....
....	....
....	....
Urinary Output	....
....	....
....	....
....	....

URINARY SYMPTOMS	Yes	No	Comments	Have they ever been clean and dry or age at onset of symptoms?
Frequency How often are they passing urine?	☐	☐		
Urge Incontinence Do they wet before reaching the toilet?	☐	☐		
Dysuria Is it painful to pass urine?	☐	☐		
Nocturia Are they woken by the urge to pass urine?	☐	☐		**Extent of wetting** ☐ 1. Damp ☐ 2. Wet - pads, pants, bed sheets
Nocturnal Enuresis Do they wet the bed?	☐	☐		☐ 3. Soaking - exterior clothes, furniture, puddle on floor, bed sheet needs changing.
Poor Stream It is a gush or a trickle?	☐	☐		
Post Micturitional Dribbling Do they leak as soon as they have finished?	☐	☐		**Behaviour prior to micturition** ☐ 1. Aggressive ☐ 2. Agitated
Lack of Sensation Does the bladder empty without warning?	☐	☐		☐ 3. Wandering ☐ 4. Pacing
Stress Incontinence When coughing, exertion, etc?	☐	☐		☐ 5. Other, please specify:
Other symptoms eg, odour?	☐	☐		☐ 6. None observed

Menstrual history, menarche and cycle ....

....

....

BOWEL SYMPTOMS

Diet including appetite and regularity of meals

	Yes	No	Is this normal? Yes	No
Liquid stool	☐	☐	☐	☐
Pebbles	☐	☐	☐	☐
Semi-formed	☐	☐	☐	☐
Formed stool	☐	☐	☐	☐
Hard stool	☐	☐	☐	☐
Straining	☐	☐	☐	☐
Faecal incontinence	☐	☐	☐	☐
Sensation of rectal fullness	☐	☐	☐	☐
Pain on defaecation	☐	☐	☐	☐
Blood	☐	☐	☐	☐
Mucus	☐	☐	☐	☐

Any exercise ....

Behaviour associated with defaecation

☐ 1. Aggressive
☐ 2. Agitated
☐ 3. Wandering
☐ 4. Pacing
☐ 5. Other, please specify:

....

☐ 6. None observed

Skin condition

☐ 1. Sore
☐ 2. Red
☐ 3. Broken
☐ 4. None observed

Bowel pattern ....

....

....

Other ....

....

Urinalysis .... Glucose .... Ketones ....

SG .... Blood .... pH ....

Protein .... Nitrites .... Leucocytes ....

MSU ....

....

Previous methods tried eg, nappies, potty training, other, charts, etc.

....

....

....

BP .... Wt .... Ht ....

Any other relevant investigations

....

....

Baseline chart given, yes/no ....

Continued additional information ....

....

....

....

....

....

....

....

Date of medical examination ....

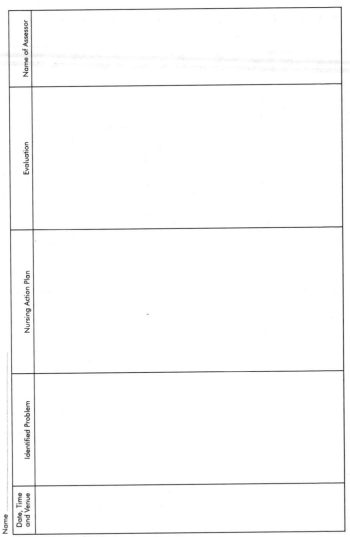

Figure 3.1A–D Children's Continence Assessment Form. Reproduced with kind permission of Nottingham Primary Care NHS Trusts.

they will ever gain control of their bowels. It may be appropriate to ascertain the views of the school. As many children attending school have problems during the day, staff have to deal with the child and the situation as and when it arises. The school may have facilities to enable the child to wash and change clothing, but in smaller schools, particularly primary schools, there is limited accommodation and this is more difficult to arrange. In some cases, the staff toilets are used because they are the only area available that will help to maintain the child's privacy and dignity. The child's social circle at school may be very limited because of the soiling problem. The noxious odours emanating from a child who soils can have a devastating effect on the child's ability to form and keep friendships, as they can keep even the most loyal supporter at bay.

On the assessment form (see Fig. 3.1A) there is a space to record details of washing facilities at home, as this is an important aspect of dealing with this condition. Information on how the family currently deals with the soiled clothing is useful too.

MEDICAL HISTORY

The medical history (page 2 of the assessment form—see Fig. 3.1B) gives an opportunity to discuss the child's general health, together

---

Box 3.1 Questions to be asked

- Age
- Date of birth
- Address
- Telephone number
- General practitioner
- School/Nursery
- Who else lives at home?
- Does the child share a bedroom?
- Does he/she share a bed?
- Does the family have access to washing machine and/or dryer at home?
- Have there been any family events that may have upset the child recently e.g. separation of parents, bereavement, house moved or new baby born etc.?
- Does anyone else in the family have a problem with their bowels?
- What is the child's normal bedtime routine?
- To the parent: What do you see as the biggest problem?
- To the child: How do you feel about your problem? Does it make you happy or sad? Would you like to stop?
- Does the school have any problems dealing with his/her condition?

with their developmental history. It should be remembered at this point that drugs used to treat some medical conditions may have an effect on the child's continence. Iron therapy is well known for either constipating the patient or giving diarrhoea, although the former is more frequently noted. If the child takes anticonvulsant drugs they may have a sedative effect and slow down gut motility. Other drugs may have base substances that affect the bladder or bowel. The family should be asked about herbal, over-the-counter and traditional medications too, as some of these may contain caffeine or have diuretic or constipating effects.

It is vital to examine factors which can impact on the child's ability to maintain continence. Mobility and dexterity are two basic skills needed to maintain continence. So information about whether the child is able to get to the toilet and if he can rearrange his clothing once there, or if the child is reliant on someone else to get him there and remove clothing as appropriate is vital. Does he have sufficient understanding to recognise the signals his body is sending and if so does he know what he should do when he gets to the toilet? Is he at the correct age developmentally?

The mechanisms and close interactions of muscle groups to facilitate voiding and defecation can be complex and it is not a skill that is usually taught. Children tend to learn by watching someone else rather than having the process described in minute detail. If the child has never had the opportunity to observe a parent on the toilet are they supposed to learn by osmosis? In some families having a child, even a very young one, observing or being close to a parent on the toilet is not considered acceptable.

Fluid intake

An investigation of fluid intake and urinary output can give an indication of areas in need of attention. The amount of fluid drunk

---

Box 3.2 Questions to be asked

- Does the child have any other medical condition?
- Does he/she have to take any medicines?
- Do you give him/her any tablets or medicines you buy yourself over the counter? Are any herbal medicines given?
- Did he/she meet all the developmental milestones when they were expected to, for example smiling, walking and talking?

Box 3.3   Questions to be asked:

- Take me through your day thinking about what you drink and how much.
- Do you have a drink with breakfast or instead of breakfast?
- What and how much do you drink? Half a cup, a large cup, a mug or just a few sips?
- Do you have another drink before you go to school or nursery?
- Again, what and how much?
- Do you have a drink mid-morning?
- If yes, what and how much?
- Do you drink with your lunch?
- What about mid-afternoon?
- What about late afternoon and evening?
- When do you have your last drink?
- What time is bedtime?

---

by the child can contribute to the problem, so investigating this closely is important. The child can be asked to list drinks taken during the day, starting from first thing in the morning.

It is important to clarify the volume and type of drink—caffeine-containing drinks should not form too high a proportion of their fluid intake: these include tea, coffee, cocoa and cola. Table 3.1 demonstrates how the optimum fluid intake can be calculated. Sufficient fluid intake is needed not only to help form and maintain a soft stool but also for renal health. Many people fail to realise the benefits of drinking sufficient fluid to help avoid constipation. A man in his sixties, who suffered longstanding constipation, once told me that he drank 'a fair amount'. When I asked him how much fluid that meant, he replied two or three glasses a day and was shocked when I suggested that a 'fair amount' was probably nearer six to eight glasses daily. It is probably fair to say

Table 3.1   Daily fluid requirements

Age	ml/kg/day
0–3 months	150
4–6 months	130
7–9 months	120
10–12 months	110
1–3 years	95
4–6 years	85
7–10 years	75
11–14 years	55
15–18 years	50

that a large proportion of the adult population does not drink the recommended levels of fluid during a day.

Urinary output

Urinary output can be ascertained in the same way as fluid intake, by asking when patients go to the toilet during the day. Can they last from break to break, if the child attends school? Urinary symptoms are often present in the child with chronic functional constipation and soiling. The large mass of faeces can occupy the space the bladder needs to expand to hold a 'normal' volume of urine. It may also irritate the bladder, causing symptoms of detrusor instability. Whitehead (1983) states: '40% of encopretics have the additional problem of enuresis.' Blethyn et al (1995) in a study of 61 children with urinary tract infection 'confirmed that faecal loading, and thus constipation, is a significant problem in children with recurrent UTI.' Vera Loening-Baucke (1997) also noted:

Relief of constipation resulted in disappearance of daytime urinary incontinence in 89% and night time urinary incontinence in 63% of patients, and a disappearance of recurrent urinary tract infections in all patients who had no anatomical abnormality of the urinary tract.

This confirms the importance of questions on urinary symptoms but the parents may need convincing by a full explanation. The use of a simple anatomical diagram to show the parent the close proximity of the bladder and bowel and how they impact upon each other can help their understanding.

Menstruation

The presence of a section on menarche and menstrual history (see Fig. 3.1B), although relevant to few clients, is important as the trigone in the bladder—the area between the ureters and urethra—

Box 3.4 Questions to be asked

- You've told me about drinking, what about when you have a wee?
- Are you wet when you wake?
- Do you use the toilet when you get up?
- Do you have to go again before leaving the house?
- Can you last until mid-morning—i.e. morning or first break, milk time etc.?

- Can you then last till lunch time, or do you have to go again?
- Do you go before and after lunch?
- Can you last till mid-afternoon or do you have to go again?
- Can you last till the end of the school day?
- Do you have to hurry home?
- How long can you then wait before needing to go again?
- How many times do you go in the evening?
- Do you remember to go before bed?
- Do you go straight to sleep?
- Do you get up to use the toilet before you go to sleep?

Asking these questions helps you to assess frequency and urgency as well as nocturnal enuresis and nocturia.
You still need to ask:

- Do you ever not make it to the toilet before you wee?
- Does it hurt when you wee?
- Do you ever have to strain when you wee?
- Do you ever wee when you didn't know you wanted to wee?
- Does the wee ever smell very strong or different?

is very sensitive to oestrogen and symptoms can therefore be more problematic at certain stages of the menstrual cycle.

Soiling history or bowel assessment

Looking at the start of symptoms can be difficult but many children with chronic functional constipation are later than their peers in passing meconium as a newborn and show symptoms as babies and toddlers. While it may be easy for the mother of a young child to remember when their child passed meconium, for the mother of an older child this is not so easy to recall. One child I managed had had constipation since the age of 4 and came to see me at the age of 10; all the child's mother could remember was that this had been a constant in their lives almost since the child had been born. A milk intolerance had led to a switch to a soya milk formula as a baby. There is some cause to pause and wonder if this actually helped the constipation at the time. Iacono et al

---

Box 3.5 Questions to be asked

- Have you started your periods?
- How often do you have a period?
- How long do they last?
- Do you have more or different problems at some times in the month?

(1995), in a small research project, found that 21 of 27 children under 3 years of age who had constipation and had cow's milk protein excluded from their diet had a reduction in their symptoms of hard stool and abdominal pain. The team measured circulating immunoglobulin E and found it to be raised in 7 of the 21 children with improvements in their symptoms, so this would seem to indicate the constipation was an allergic response to the cow's milk protein. Loening-Baucke (1998) reminds us that alongside the more easily recognised allergic responses of diarrhoea and vomiting, allergic rhinitis, asthma and eczema, 'chronic constipation caused by anal erythema, anal fissures, anal fistulas and proctitis have been attributed to intolerance of cow's milk protein.' Buchanan (1992) in her text cites the work of Coekin & Gairdner in 1960 which noted 'the relationship between cow's milk, constipation and soiling.' If this was noted in the 1960s it begs the question, why has this knowledge not been used previously in the treatment of chronic functional constipation?

Feverish illness in a baby may result in constipation if the fluid lost through the raised temperature is not replaced. A small rise in temperature for a short period of time can result in constipation for those who are prone to it; a simple cold may be sufficient to cause constipation. In young babies this has a more dramatic effect than in older children and adults. The hard stool that results is painful to pass, leading to withholding which gives a harder stool as more water is reabsorbed, resulting in more pain and so the cycle goes on. Advising the mother to increase fluids at this time is vital; she should offer drinks between feeds and, if the baby is bottle-fed, adding an extra ounce of water in the feed without increasing the amount of formula.

Fig. 3.1C explores bowel symptoms, starting with the child's faeces or, in their language, 'poo'. It is important when assessing children to include them in the assessment, if possible. One way of including them in the interview is to ensure you do not exclude them by the language you use—most children think a stool is something to sit on!

You need to decide who is going to be able to give the most information about the child's faeces. For the baby and younger child, you need to address your questions to the parent but for an older child, it may be better to talk directly to the patient. Any parent of a child over 5 years of age would find it difficult to describe their child's faeces. Loening-Baucke (1997) agrees:

'It was our experience that parents paid little attention to the frequency of their child's bowel movements, but paid much attention to the number of urinary and faecal incontinence episodes.' Using a copy of the Bristol Stool Form Chart, developed by Dr Ken Heaton, can be very beneficial: the parent or child chooses the version which most resembles their own stool! (see Fig. 3.2). This scale was designed and validated with an adult population, however it appears to work as effectively with children. They appear to enjoy being able to point to a diagram rather than trying to put into words a description of their faeces.

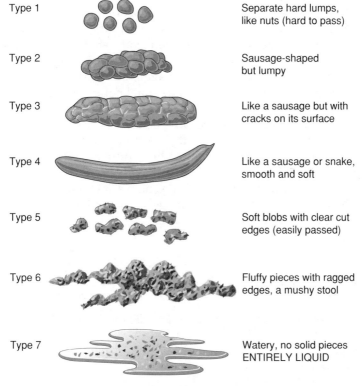

Type 1		Separate hard lumps, like nuts (hard to pass)
Type 2		Sausage-shaped but lumpy
Type 3		Like a sausage but with cracks on its surface
Type 4		Like a sausage or snake, smooth and soft
Type 5		Soft blobs with clear cut edges (easily passed)
Type 6		Fluffy pieces with ragged edges, a mushy stool
Type 7		Watery, no solid pieces ENTIRELY LIQUID

Figure 3.2 Bristol Stool Form Chart. The scale was designed and validated with an adult population. (Reproduced by kind permission of Dr KW Heaton, Reader in Medicine at the University of Bristol. Produced by Norgine Limited, manufacturers of Movicol.)

Even if unable to describe the everyday stools, many parents can give graphic accounts of the truly spectacular bowel evacuations their child has: 'It's so big it blocks the toilet' or 'You wouldn't believe someone so little could have such a big poo.' and 'It looks as if it comes from someone else it's so large.' These are frequent comments heard from parents. In between these huge evacuations the child has a few days with no problems and then starts to soil again as liquid faeces starts to seep around the growing mass and leak out. This leaking substance is exceptionally offensive as it has been 'brewing' in the colon and rectum for several days.

In addition to recording the appearance of the child's faeces, it is necessary to discover if the child is aware of the need to pass faeces and whether it is painful (and for many it is). Van der Plas et al's (1997) description of constipation and their definition of the large faecal mass passed certainly is appropriate for these children. It is necessary to record what the pattern is, how frequent, how often does the child have a huge evacuation, when does the soiling start again and what does it look like? Does the child have any abdominal pain prior to evacuation or at other times? We can use this to aid in a toiletting programme. Likewise, is there any behaviour associated with defecation? At what time do they soil or defecate? Listen to other methods tried—no matter how off-the-wall they may appear—they indicate a degree of motivation on either the child or the parent's behalf. Some of the methods tried will indicate health professional enthusiasm, including referral for investigation, laxatives etc.

Box 3.6   Questions to be asked

- When did your child first have his/her bowels open and pass meconium (the black tarry stuff all babies pass)—was it later than the other babies on the ward?
- What does the poo look like—can you find one that looks like it on this chart (Bristol Stool Chart)?
- Do you ever have to push hard to poo?
- Is it ever painful?
- Is there ever any blood in it?
- Is there ever any slime in it?
- How often do you go?
- How often does poo escape into your pants?
- What have you tried in the past to stop this happening?

Dietary assessment

The dietary intake of the whole family and particularly the child can be revealing. One child I saw briefly before his mother defaulted further appointments (she had lots of social problems and it had been difficult for her to attend even one appointment), ate only chips, burgers and sausage and baked beans. Mother claimed that she offered him other foods, particularly vegetables only to have them left on the plate and wasted. As she was receiving benefits she could not afford this. Most do make an attempt at eating some fibre but have often had little proper or professional guidance on what to eat.

Ask the child what they ate the day before at the first appointment, as this is often fairly representative of other days. A more thorough assessment is still needed and this can be gained from a food diary completed by the family. The food diary could be sent with the appointment for the first interview or given at this time to complete before their next appointment at the same time as the other baseline data are being collected. The advantage of sending it with the appointment letter is that it is available to examine and discuss at the assessment, although incorrect completion may be a problem when there has not been a full explanation. While there may be some element of bias in the completion after the first interview (parents may report what they think you want to hear, rather than being accurate), the information gained could be more useful in the long run. There is more on the role of diet in Chapter 6.

Exercise

Exercise can play a useful part in increasing gut motility, so it can be interesting to ascertain what exercise the child has outside of

---

Box 3.7 Questions to be asked

- Tell me what you had to eat yesterday.
- Start with breakfast. (What type of cereal or bread?)
- Any snack mid-morning?
- What did you have for lunch? (Again, what type of bread and/or potatoes?)
- Any snack in the afternoon?
- What did you have for the evening meal?
- Anything else before bed?

that provided by nursery/school/childminder. Kamm & Lennard-Jones (1994) tell us 'The ingestion of food and physical activity both produce an increase in colonic activity, and this consists of an increase in both segmenting and propagated contractions.' It is unusual for children with constipation and soiling to be involved in any activities apart from those that are statutory and provided by school or nursery. Whether this is an effect of the lower, though not abnormal, levels of thyroxine these children can have is uncertain (see Chapter 4). As health professionals, we should encourage activity in all children, not only to prevent constipation but also to promote their long-term health, including that of their cardiovascular system, and to improve their bone density and their mental well-being.

Behaviour

Understanding and observing behaviour associated with defecation can be useful in helping with the management of youngsters with constipation. Children with specific learning difficulties may demonstrate certain behaviour patterns, such as rocking or pacing prior to defecation. Parents and other carers can observe this and then take the child to sit on the toilet. It is rare that the child whose development is within normal limits exhibits behaviour such as this.

Skin

Skin condition in children is almost without exception good, even in children with profound learning difficulties, no mobility and poor nutritional and fluid intake. Some specialist paediatric centres may see pressure sores but they are rare. However, it is worth asking, as other problems may be mentioned, including nappy rash in the child with urinary incontinence. Nappy rash is not exclusive to nappy wearers.

Box 3.8 Questions to be asked

- Do you take part in any activities outside school, e.g. scouts, swimming club, football, etc?
- Do you go out to play after school?
- What sort of things do you do?

Box 3.9 Questions to be asked

- Have you noticed any particular behaviour associated with the desire to poo?
- Is there any problem with the child's skin?

INVESTIGATIONS

Urinalysis is important to exclude a UTI, as mentioned earlier. See Chapter 4 for a full description of urinalysis and the significance of what is identified during testing. If a dipstick urinalysis indicates the presence of protein, blood, nitrites or leucocytes, then a midstream (if possible) sample should be sent for microculture and sensitivity testing so that appropriate therapy can be commenced. Sometimes the child's blood pressure is measured and plotted against centile charts, which are height-specific, so the height and weight are measured too, (see Figs 3.3 and 3.4). There may be occasional incidences of a child with hypertension which needs investigating and treating if necessary.

Other relevant investigations include urodynamics, abdominal X-ray or for example, a rectal biopsy to exclude Hirschsprung's disease. If baseline data have not already been collected, ensure this is done now.

SOILING DETAILS

Most of the information collected so far is essential for the treatment of any continence problem in a child. However, there is specific information required to assess chronic functional constipation with overflow soiling. Whether the child has ever had control of their bowels has already been asked but it is worth getting finer details on this. Closer questioning can be used as follows:

1. Does the child soil every day or are there some days when he doesn't soil?

Box 3.10 Questions to be asked

- What tests, if any, have been done before to check what causes your problem? (MSU, X-ray, blood tests or biopsy?)

Height-Specific Blood Pressure Percentiles
BOYS

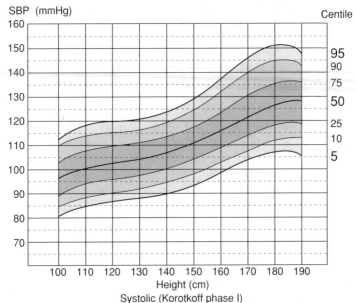

Systolic (Korotkoff phase I)

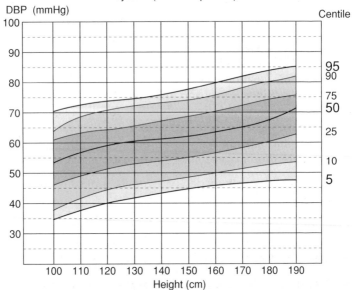

Diastolic (Korotkoff phase V)

Figure 3.3 Boys' Blood Pressure Centile Chart.

Height-Specific Blood Pressure Percentiles
GIRLS

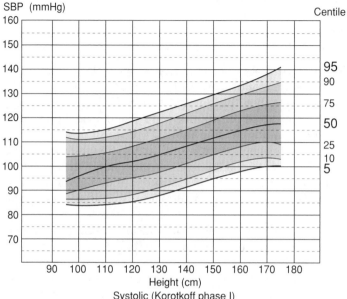

Systolic (Korotkoff phase I)

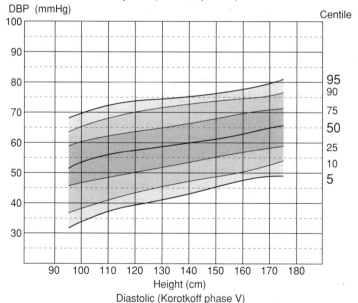

Diastolic (Korotkoff phase V)

Figure 3.4 Girls' Blood Pressure Centile Chart.

2. Is there a pattern to this?
3. Following a large evacuation, or on particular days of the week, does the child pass a reasonably normal stool at any time? If so, what happens to start the problem again?
4. Perhaps even more important and interesting is: What happens to cause the normal stool?

Make a record of instances of soiling, including the timing, e.g. after meals, time of day, events leading to the soiling and where the child was when the soiling happened. If the soiling occurs after meals it can be incorporated in a management programme. Requesting that the child be allowed time to sit on the toilet after a meal when the gastrocolic reflex is at its strongest can engender success. This is easier if the reflex is happening when the child is at home. If the child gets a gastrocolic reflex at all, even if at inconvenient times or in difficult places, we can try to reproduce it at other times.

Has the child had a recent and relevant medical examination, including an abdominal examination/palpation? Unfortunately, this is not always conclusive as the faeces accumulating in the higher sections of the colon are often soft and therefore not palpated as loaded colon. (Many people associate constipation with the hardness of the stool, not with the delay of passage of stool.) Has the anus been examined to exclude fissures or any other abnormality? Has blood been taken for thyroid function tests to exclude hypothyroidism?

SOCIAL RELATIONSHIPS

Invest time in exploring family relationships: is there one particular member of the family with whom the child has a good relationship? Can this be the person to support the child through his management programme? Don't forget this means long-term support of over a year for the longer-standing problem.

Box 3.11 Questions to be asked

- Does the child soil every day?
- Is there a pattern?
- Does he ever pass a normal stool?
- At what time of day does the soiling occur?
- Does it happen after meals?

Conversely, is there a relationship which is not good and cre-
ates antagonism which may hinder the management programme? The child needs to have positive support during what
can be a very trying time for the whole family. As a health professional, you must reward the person supporting the child with
praise at every appointment. Tell them how hard they are working and how much this is contributing to the child's success.

The child's relationships with his peers are also an important
aspect of his life and therefore should not be ignored during
assessment. The child aged over 5 years spends many hours
every day at school, so involving staff at the school can be beneficial. Perhaps a 'circle of friends' could be set up to support the
child at school. This concept involves the recruitment of children
from the patient's class to help to remind the child, in this case,
when to go to the toilet to get cleaned up.

One difficulty with this is, as mentioned earlier, that the child's
faeces smell abominably and getting another child or children to
stay close and give support can be very difficult. All children can
be very cruel if a child is any different from the others; a child
who smells can be a great target for them. The taunting and isolation which can follow can further reduce the child's self-esteem.
In a large school, there may be more than one child suffering and
these children may form a support system for each other. This is
far from ideal as their own self-esteem is too low to form positive
support for another child with the same condition. Staff at school
are only human and many find they are disgusted by a child who
has no bowel control. Many will find that nursery and school staff
have a very negative attitude towards the condition. Liaison with
these members of staff either directly yourself or through the
child's health visitor or school nurse to explain the problem fully
and help them work through their anxieties is essential.

Practical considerations such as working out who will help the
child clean up and change clothing, where the soiled clothing can
be stored, when parents will be informed, etc. are helpful. As a
health professional, you also need to consider whether advice on
Hepatitis B immunisation is appropriate for staff and who will
administer the vaccine if necessary. Should the education or social
services occupational health department be involved and organise a session to immunise all staff involved, do they attend their
own GP and, if so, who pays for the prescription charges? Can
they claim from petty cash or do they have to pay their own

charges? These are some of the questions that may arise so it might be worthwhile investigating the situation locally so you are prepared if any queries arise. You also need to consider whether you are prepared, if asked, to administer the vaccine yourself if necessary. Is there a protocol or is a patient group directive available for this situation? If not, is one needed, as the situation is likely to arise again?

ABUSE

When assessing a child you must always remain alert to signs of abuse, both physical as punishment for soiling and sexual abuse. Buchanan (1992) states:

> Experience suggests that there may be three possible triggers for soiling following sexual abuse. Firstly fine bowel control may be damaged by buggery; secondly the post trauma of the assault may trigger psychological mechanisms resulting in soiling; and thirdly some of the children may use soiling as a defence against unwanted sexual advances.

Although it is necessary to be mindful of a serious problem we must balance the protection of the child with the need to avoid misdiagnosis. We have all seen the high-profile cases in the past where the over-diagnosis of sexual abuse has helped no-one at all.

RESPONSES

We need to establish the level of the child's motivation. How do they feel about what happens to them? Many youngsters who have tried different methods but for insufficient time-spans often feel it is rather hopeless and they will never regain control over their bowels. Part of the health professional's role

---

Box 3.12 Questions to be asked

- Whom does the child get on well with?
- Who helps the child to clean up?
- Is there someone who doesn't help?
- Does the child have a special friend or friends?
- If the child is school-aged, who helps at school?
- What happens—is there a special toilet?
- What happens to the soiled clothing?

is to dispel this feeling, but it will not happen at one visit; constant effort is required to raise morale and motivation at each visit. Record what the child has tried, but remember there will often be a list of the methods tried over the months and years of this condition. Explore the benefits to the child of gaining bowel control. Ask what the problem prevents the child from doing. For most children and young people social activities can be seriously curtailed. Examine the parental response to soiling:

1. Is there anger, and if so what punishments does the anger lead to?
2. Does this warrant being referred as a child protection issue?
3. Can you refer and still work comfortably with the family to manage the child's constipation, or would it be better for a colleague to take over? There needs to be a degree of trust between the family and the health professional if they are to comply with the management you advise.
4. If no anger is displayed, do the parents exhibit disgust? How can you deal with this? There is no easy answer to this; some people will always find it difficult to deal with, but a full explanation can help a little. Informing the parents that the child does not soil deliberately, as some think, can help.
5. How do the parents deal with episodes of soiling?
6. Are there arrangements in place for the child to deal with dirty clothing?
7. Is the child praised on days when soiling does not occur or when the toilet is used successfully? *All of these little pieces of information help to form a more complete picture of what is happening and the management required.*
8. How does the child respond to the soiling?
9. Does the child acknowledge it, or remain unaware it has happened?
10. Does the child deny it has happened even when the soiling is apparent to everyone around?
11. How does the child react when told to clean up and change?
12. Does the child display anger or shame?
13. Does the child hide soiled underwear; if so, where would the parents prefer the soiled clothing to be placed?

This can be the start of a management programme.

An accurate description of the size and consistency of the faeces should be obtained. While the Bristol Stool Form Chart can help with the consistency, the size can be more difficult to ascertain. There are clay models that can demonstrate the varying sizes of faeces passed which may be useful. If there is no access to the professional sets, can a set be made either with modelling clay or self-hardening clay?

Try to explore the child's attempts to defecate. Have the parents ever watched? Probably not, in most cases. Do you need to explain the defecation process (see Chapter 2)? Are there ways it can be made easier for the child? Bonner, a continence advisor in Luton, has developed a whistle-like instrument that children use when attempting to defecate. This encourages them to blow, rather than hold their breath, during the process. Ask parents to watch the child and make a mental note of the information required.

Does the child even sit on the toilet? Or has this never been attempted because insufficient bowel control has meant the patient still wears nappies? A four-year-old in my caseload was still in nappies and staff at nursery noticed that when he had the urge to defecate he squatted wherever he was and started to soil his nappy. This situation is far from ideal and should be stopped immediately. In this case the staff stopped him and took him to the toilets where he then continued to soil his nappy. Perhaps toilet training had not been a priority in the family and they had taken the easy option of leaving the child in nappies. What laxatives had they tried, in what order and for how long?

Many health professionals do not realise that the child needs medication for long periods of time, so when first contacting the child's GP, advance notice should be given that treatment will be needed for perhaps up to 2 years. Many health professionals are also not aware of the need for different types of laxatives and the fact that different doses are required at different stages of treatment. Does the child take any other medication on a regular basis? If so, what is it, and will it have an effect on the child's bowels—is there an alternative? What stimulates a gastrocolic reflex in the child; can this be tried again and produce the same response every time? Have the family noted any particular foodstuff or drink that affects the child's bowel movements? Do you have a list of ideas? (see Chapter 7).

Box 3.13   Questions to be asked

- How do you feel about your problem?
- Would you like to stop?
- Have you tried anything previously to help your problem—what was it and did it work?
- What else will change when you no longer have your problem?
- Does your problem stop you doing some things—if so, what?
- As a parent, how do you feel about the problem?
- What do you say or do when your child has an accident?
- How do you cope with the accident?
- Is there an agreed place where your child puts soiled clothing?
- What do you say or do on days when there is no soiling or when the child uses the toilet successfully?
- Ask the child—what do you do when you have an accident?
- Do you know when it has happened? Every time?
- Does someone have to tell you it has happened?
- Where do you put your soiled clothing?
- Have you ever watched your child trying to poo?
- Does your child sit on the toilet or still wear nappies?
- Have you tried any medicines/laxatives before?
- Which ones?
- Can you remember how much and how often each one was taken and for how long?
- Does the child take any other medicines or tablets at all?
- Does the child have tummy pain before pooing?
- Does the child poo after eating or drinking?

BASELINE DATA COLLECTION

Whilst much of the baseline data can be gathered during the initial interview with the child and the child's family, other information needs to be collected by the family between this visit and subsequent appointments.

A fluid balance type chart should also be issued (see Fig. 3.5) Although it is simple, it is easy to complete, which improves the chance of compliance. Each day has a column for drinks taken and another for voiding, either by wetting or using the toilet. If you require more detailed information ask the parent to write 'glass' or 'cup' in the drinks column. Most parents are also willing to measure the urine voided for a couple of days, using a jug, and record it on the chart. (Find out where these can be purchased locally for very little expense unless your employer will provide them. There is a large chain of hardware stores that sells them for less than 50 pence.)

A food diary kept for a minimum of four days is essential; looking at each meal and the snacks the child, and the family, take can be enlightening and useful later in their treatment.

Fluid Balance Chart.

Please complete this chart accurately. Tick the first column each time a drink is taken and the second column when urine is passed. Name_____

Date_____

Time	Mon	Mon	Tues	Tues	Wed	Wed	Thur	Thur	Fri	Fri	Sat	Sat	Sun	Sun
7am														
8am														
9am														
10am														
11am														
12am														
1pm														
2pm														
3pm														
4pm														
5pm														
6pm														
7pm														
8pm														
9pm														
10pm														
11pm														
12pm														
1am														
2am														
3am														
4am														
5am														
6am														
Totals														

Figure 3.5 Fluid Balance Chart.

A soiling chart (see Fig. 3.6) can be issued too. Decide what information is required; the chart shown in Figure 3.9 gives the necessary information in a succinct format. You may consider a structured interview with the child which would include the following questions:

Soiling Baseline Chart					
Day	used toilet	soiled	other symptoms	laxatives taken softener:	and times stimulant:
Monday					
Tuesday					
Wednesday					
Thursday					
Friday					
Saturday					
Sunday					
Monday					
Tuesday					
Wednesday					
Thursday					
Friday					
Saturday					
Sunday					
Monday					
Tuesday					
Wednesday					
Thursday					
Friday					
Saturday					
Sunday					

Figure 3.6 Soiling Baseline Chart.

1. Do they know what to do? Do they have the sensation of the need to defecate, can they coordinate the muscular activity required to defecate? (Do you know how to poo? Does your body tell you when you need a poo?)
2. Do they wish to cooperate in changing their soiling behaviour? (Do you want to do something to help stop the poo escaping into your pants?)
3. Do they recognise the benefit of being in control of their bowels? (What will change if the poo does not escape any more?)
4. Does soiling interfere with their lifestyle? (Does the poo escaping stop you doing things?)
5. How does the child feel others view the problem? (What do other people think about your poo escaping?)

Baseline information should be collected for between 2 and 4 weeks with no intervention. It is vital, because collecting accurate baseline data should result in finding out exactly what the child is able and unable to do, so you can decide what it is the child needs. You will then be able to design a programme to meet those needs. It also provides an opportunity to compare and contrast the child's progress against the baseline situation as the management proceeds. *Do not forget assessment is an ongoing process.*

REFERENCES

Blethyn A J, Jenkins H R, Roberts R, Jones K Verrier 1995 Radiological evidence of constipation in urinary tract infection. Archives of Disease in Childhood 73(6): 534–535
Buchanan A 1992 Children who soil: assessment and treatment. John Wiley, Chichester
Iacono G, Carroccio A, Cavataio F, Montalto G, Cantarero M D, Notarbartolo A 1995 Chronic constipation as a symptom of cow milk allergy. The Journal of Pediatrics 126(1): 34–39
Kamm M A, Lennard-Jones J E (eds) 1994 Constipation. Wrightston Biomedical Publishing, Petersfield
Loening-Baucke V 1997 Urinary incontinence and urinary tract infection and their resolution with treatment of chronic constipation of childhood. Pediatrics 100(2): 228–232
Loening-Baucke V 1998 Constipation in children (Editorial) The New England Journal of Medicine 339(16): 1155–1156
van der Plas R N, Benninga M A, Redekop W K, Taminiau J A, Buller H A 1997 How accurate is the recall of bowel habits in children with defaecation disorders? European Journal of Pediatrics 156: 178–181
Whitehead N 1983 Childhood encopresis—a clinical psychologist's approach. Health Visitor 56(Sep): 335–336

4

Specific tests

Urinalysis	Leucocytes
Glucose	Blood tests
Ketones	Abdominal X-ray
Specific gravity	Marker studies
Blood	Rectal manometry
pH	Barium enema
Protein	Rectal biopsy
Nitrite	

Although a thorough history is vital to establish an effective programme of therapeutic intervention to help the children and young people who suffer chronic functional constipation with overflow soiling, there are also specific tests which can help to complete the picture painted by that assessment. Some of the tests can only be carried out in specialist centres or by hospital services but, where possible, some easier versions are suggested here. The availability of some of the investigations described will depend upon whether there is a local paediatrician who has an interest in the children. In Chapter 3, some of the basic investigations which can be carried out on all children and young people with continence problems have been listed; a more detailed description follows here.

URINALYSIS

Urinalysis is one of the basic tests that all nurses are taught during their training, but in how much detail? While children, like adults, can have asymptomatic bacteriuria, there is an increased risk of urinary tract infection in the presence of chronic constipation. Some of this will be due to the seepage of liquid or semi-formed faeces from the anus, and some due to the fact that the anus may be partially open at all times, with a faecal mass in the anal canal. Both of these situations result in common gut bacteria being present in the anogenital area, allowing easy access to the urinary tract, and thus the infection becomes established. Blethyn et al (1995a) found that between 38% and 54% of the children they studied who had had between 1 and more than 5 previous urinary tract infections (UTI) had some degree of faecal loading on abdominal X-ray. They gave some suggestions for the cause of UTI with constipation, citing other works that note an interrelationship between constipation and urinary tract abnormalities. The faecal mass is thought to act as a mechanical cause of distortion of the bladder and urethra, and possibly results in the inability to completely empty the bladder, leading to a residual volume of urine at risk of bacterial infection. They demonstrated, as others have done, that the aggressive treatment of the constipation helped with the treatment of the urinary symptoms.

Let us consider what we are looking for when we carry out a routine urinalysis and what we should do with the results. There are different types of testing strip on the market and each health service provider will have its own favoured product. However, all have a similar function, namely to identify any abnormalities in the clients' urine that needs either more sensitive testing or other investigations.

Preparation for testing is important and should also involve advising clients on specimen collection. Ideally, this should be an early morning sample, but this is not always possible as it is often collected at the clinic session due to the impracticality of sending a clean bottle to the home with the appointment. The child should, if possible, void directly either into a sterile sample bottle or into a clean dry receptacle which should be labelled if at all possible. The urine should be tested as soon as possible as changes will occur in the specimen if it is left exposed to light and heat. If it is collected significantly in advance of the clinic it should be refrigerated and brought back to room temperature before testing, which should be done within 4 hours of it being produced.

The first aspect of testing is to consider the appearance and smell of the urine collected. Is it cloudy or clear, what colour is it, is the smell offensive? These factors will be noticed almost subconsciously but they form a vital part of the urine testing procedure.

Bayer Diagnostics (undated) give some detailed information on urinalysis, but the following is the information relevant to the condition described in this text. It is of the utmost importance to follow the manufacturer's instructions carefully when using testing strips so these should have been read and understood before the test is carried out. All of the reagent areas should be fully immersed in the urine briefly; the strip should then be removed from the urine and the side of the strip should be wiped along the rim of the container to remove any drips. The strip must then be kept horizontal to prevent the different chemicals from mixing and the time should be measured before each reagent area is compared with the result chart provided at the appropriate times. Keeping the strip horizontal also helps to prevent contamination of the clinician's hand.

What should the urine be tested for routinely in a clinic for children with constipation and soiling? There are a number of different substances which can be tested by reagent strip. Some, while not specific to the client group, are included on the test strip anyway, others should be considered because of the benefit to the client if other conditions are indicated.

Glucose

Glucose is one such test as it is often included on test strips, but it would obviously be remiss of any health professional to ignore any abnormality in this test. Glucose is found in the urine of individuals when its levels in the plasma are higher than the renal threshold. The commonest cause of glucose in the urine is diabetes mellitus, so any child found to have glucose in the urine should be referred back to his general practitioner for further investigations.

Ketones

The presence of ketones in the urine is usually an indication that body fat is being broken down. In adults, this may be due to dieting, but in children it is often due to fasting, or diarrhoea and vomiting, but can also indicate poorly controlled insulin-dependent diabetes. Please remember that although younger children are exempt, Muslims fast during Ramadan and therefore older Muslim children may have ketonuria at this time, especially if they are seen late in the day.

Specific gravity

This is an indication of the amount of solutes in the urine, so very concentrated urine will have a higher reading than very dilute urine. The values vary naturally in healthy patients so, unless the values are widely outside those indicated on the result chart, it is of little use clinically.

Blood

This indicates the presence of whole red blood cells, or haemoglobin, in the urine. This often indicates either renal problems or infection of the urinary tract but can less commonly indicate a sickle cell crisis, a metabolic disorder or other rare conditions. Infection should be excluded as a first measure before other more detailed tests are carried out by the general practitioner or paediatrician.

pH

This measures the acidity or alkalinity of a solution. In a healthy individual the normal range for urine is between 4.5 and 8.0, dependent on the kidneys' ability to eliminate hydrogen ions. The level can be changed by an infection with organisms containing an enzyme which increases the amount of ammonia produced from urea. Common causes of low values are diabetic ketoacidosis, starvation, and potassium depletion. High values are commonly caused by stale urine, but in fresh urine they may be due to vomiting or taking large volumes of antacids, or urinary tract infection with the ammonia-forming organisms mentioned.

Protein

Most often the test strips indicate the presence of albumin which is in the urine because the membranes of the glomeruli are more permeable than normal. It is not an indicator of infection.

Nitrite

This substance is found in the urine only when there is an infection, particularly by organisms which convert nitrate to nitrite.

Nitrate is normally found in the urine. Not all microorganisms will convert nitrate to nitrite, so a negative result for nitrite does not necessarily exclude the presence of urinary infection.

Leucocytes

Leucocytes are white blood cells found in the body in high concentration when there is an infection. In urinary tract infections some of these leucocytes will pass through inflamed tissues into the urine. The inflamed tissue is usually present when there is an acute infection.

BLOOD TESTS

Perhaps the most common screen carried out when blood testing children and young people with chronic constipation and soiling is to test thyroid function. Hypothyroidism is a common cause of constipation in both adults and children and is easily excluded on testing. Stern et al (1995) found that, although within normal limits, thyroxine levels in children with soiling were lower than control children not suffering from soiling with chronic constipation.

For the children seen at local clinics this is the only routine test required. However, Stern et al (1995) also tested for and compared levels of other circulating hormones affecting the gastrointestinal tract. They were particularly interested in those that altered the motility of the gastrointestinal tract. They took blood samples from a small group of children with constipation and soiling and a group of controls matched for age, race and gender at different times throughout one day. They tested for levels of pancreatic polypeptide, gastrin, cholecystokinin and motilin as well as oestrogen and thyroxine. As a control they tested insulin levels, as it is a gastrointestinal hormone but one with no effect on the gut motility. The blood samples were taken twice (20 and 5 minutes) before and ten times after (at intervals varying between 5 and 180 minutes) a liquid meal replacement was given. The results showed that there were differences in the plasma levels of the hormones that affect gastrointestinal motility between the two groups of children, with some being significant and others not so. The main differences were demonstrated after the meal replacement was given.

It appears from this research, then, that children with chronic constipation and soiling have a physiological reason for their condition. Motilin increases both gastric and small intestine motility and plays a role in the peristaltic movement of the contents through the small intestine to empty into the colon, and in these children the level was lower. They were found to have higher post-prandial levels of pancreatic polypeptide which has been demonstrated to be associated with lower levels of motilin. The variation in the levels of the cholecystokinin were not found to be significant, although they were slightly lower in the constipated children. As this hormone affects motility of the colon, it may also have a role to play in the condition. These tests are not, however, routine tests and perhaps should never become so but do help to explain what may be exacerbating the condition.

ABDOMINAL X-RAY

While X-rays are more commonly used to identify bony abnormalities, they can demonstrate faecal impaction very clearly. This may be important in giving affected children and their families a visual insight into the condition. They are perhaps also useful in that the faecal loading of the colon may involve soft faeces which may be missed on abdominal palpation. Blethyn et al (1995b) devised a scoring system for abdominal X-ray on children who were constipated, from Grade 0, where the normal situation is found with faeces in the caecum and rectum only, through to Grade 3, where there are excessive amounts of faeces in the caecum and rectum with some elsewhere in the colon which is dilated and there is an impacted rectum. In the study, 6 observers—two of them experienced and four less experienced in paediatrics—individually assessed 20 abdominal radiographs and gave them a score from the grading system. They found there was a high number of agreements on the grade given and, in those where there was disagreement, there was only one grade difference in most, with a small number of two-grade differences. The team felt they had devised a good grading system for assessing children's chronic constipation, particularly where the clinical history is confused. Many authors, including this team, agree:

that we would certainly not advocate the use of an abdominal radiograph to diagnose most cases of constipation but, in certain circumstances it may be useful, occasionally when it is difficult to tell clinically whether constipation is present and, more especially, to obtain retrospective evidence of faecal loading.

Many units do not carry out abdominal radiographs even when severe constipation is present; local policy should be investigated to ascertain the reasons for this. It may be due to a lack of a scoring or grading system or disagreement with the usefulness of X-ray in this condition, or it may be because of concern for the levels of radiation despite there being a low level of exposure during this particular investigation. There are, however, tests that could combine two different investigations that require an abdominal X-ray.

MARKER STUDIES

This is a method of assessing the gastrocolic transit times of children with severe or chronic constipation. In this test, children are asked to swallow a number of radioopaque polyethylene pellets on day one. These are usually approximately 2, 3 or 5 mm in diameter and come in different shapes. While the most simple test would involve giving one batch of these and taking an abdominal X-ray between 24–72 hours later to see how far the pellets have progressed, it can be refined. Refined versions of the transit time studies involve giving different-shaped markers at daily intervals for 3 days and taking an X-ray on day five. This gives a more complete picture of how the pellets are progressing through the gas-trointestinal tract. Lennard-Jones (Kamm & Lennard-Jones 1994) discusses transit studies at some length. He cites work done in 1985 by Corazziari et al, who studied 78 children with no bowel problems aged between 2 months and 12 years and found that 80% of the markers were passed within 19 to 33 hours. However, when they compared these results with children complaining of chronic constipation, they found that 53 out of 63 had prolonged transit time, although these times fell within normal adult times. If there are worries about exposing children to radioactivity, it is possible to X-ray the stools passed when conducting these studies, although obviously this needs careful planning for collection and handling of specimens.

If these tests are not available to you a 'Heath Robinson' method may be tried, where the child is fed sweetcorn and the mother makes a note of how long after ingestion this is seen in the stool. Sweetcorn is an ideal substance to use as it is very visible in the stool and appears little changed; it is also palatable to most children and it is therefore usually fairly easy to persuade them to eat it. Obviously, this version of the test, while easily undertaken, can only give the total transit time, whereas the more clinical tests give indications of precisely where the slower transit occurs.

RECTAL MANOMETRY

This test is rarely carried out on children in the UK, but is used on adults. In many other countries, the test is an expected part of the history and assessment of children with chronic constipation and is therefore more routine. Getliffe & Dolman (1997) tell us: 'The tests measure the effectiveness and strength of the anal sphincters, together with the degree of sensation felt within the rectum.' Here it is reserved primarily for excluding Hirschsprung's disease, as the rectoanal inhibitory reflex is absent on the measurements recorded during the test. Clayden & Agnarsson (1991) suggest the test should be carried out ideally without sedation, the patient should not be faecally loaded and should have received no enemata, suppositories or manual evacuation of faeces within the previous 3 days. The child should not have been given any stimulant laxatives for 36 hours prior to the procedure.

The child is prepared and taken to the examination room and asked to lie on their left side. A probe is then inserted into the patient's rectum via the anal canal (see Fig. 4.1A). There are a number of different probes available and various techniques are used to carry out the test. Kamm (1994) tells us: 'Anal manometry can be performed using a variety of techniques, including a closed microballoon air or water filled system, a perfused side hole catheter, or a solid state strain gauge system.'

Once the probe is in the correct position (see Fig. 4.1B), the balloon is inflated and anal and rectal pressures are recorded, together with any relaxation or contraction of the internal and external anal sphincters. The recordings should demonstrate the relaxation of the internal sphincter and the simultaneous contraction of the external anal sphincter, as the rectum and anal canal become accustomed to the presence of the balloon and a reduction in anal pressure is noted. Several authors, including Loening-Baucke (in Kamm 1994), have performed these tests and compared children with and without chronic constipation, and children with Hirschsprung's disease.

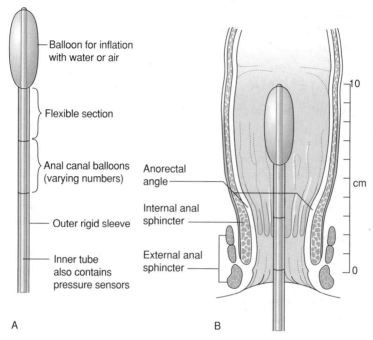

A

B

Figure 4.1A,B Anorectal probe and its position during the test.

Children with no bowel problems were found to have a drop in anal pressure, as were those with chronic constipation, but those with Hirschsprung's did not demonstrate this. The volumes required to stimulate this reflex and cause the drop in anal pressure are much smaller in the normal healthy child than in the constipated child. Further tests were done to elicit the minimum volume in the balloon required to precipitate a lasting urge to defecate, termed the 'critical volume' by the author. To do this, the balloon was inflated in stages of 10 ml of air, until it contained 60 ml. It was then inflated in 30-ml stages, until there was constant relaxation of both internal and external sphincters. In a control group of healthy children this volume was approximately 90 ml. In 'a child with chronic constipation and faecal soiling with mild impairment of rectal sensation and rectal contractility' the volume required was approximately 180 ml. In 'a child with chronic constipation and faecal soiling with severe impairment in rectal sensation and rectal contractility, indicating rectal atony,' the volume required was approximately 330 ml. This is more than three times the volume a normal healthy child requires and gives an indication of the size of stool these children pass occasionally (Fig. 4.2).

BARIUM ENEMA

Many health professionals will have seen the results of barium enemata and may have accompanied patients undergoing them. For those who are not aware of the nature of these examinations, barium enemata can be undertaken to outline the size of the rectum and colon. They are performed on severely constipated children who have functional problems. As the pictures will clearly illustrate the size of the rectum, they are useful in the assessment of Hirschsprung's disease and other neurogenic conditions of the large intestine.

The patient is usually given one or two doses of sodium picosulfate to empty the colon and rectum the night prior to the examination. They should, however, be advised that it may result in abdominal cramps and dehydration as it decreases water absorption from the colon, small amount though this is. Food intake is limited, but the child should be allowed to drink as much as he wants, especially to counteract the fluid loss mentioned earlier. When the child arrives in the X-ray department, an enema of barium is administered and the child is asked to move into different positions to coat the colon with the medium. When this has been achieved, the radiographs are taken while the child lies on a moving couch. The barium is then expelled. More X-rays may be required at this time. The procedure is not comfortable and should be explained as fully as possible to the child at a level appropriate to his understanding.

Barium can also have constipating effects so, with the effects of previous possible dehydration from the sodium picosulfate, it is vital that the parents are advised to encourage an increased fluid intake to try to avoid further problems.

RECTAL BIOPSY

This is carried out in order to obtain histological and histochemical information. It is a test done primarily to exclude or diagnose Hirschsprung's disease or other neurogenic disorders. It should be carried out by a skilled paediatric surgeon,

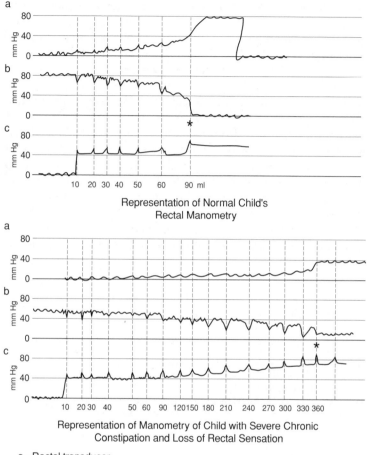

a - Rectal transducer

b - Anal transducer

c - Rectal balloon

★ - Constant relaxation

Figure 4.2 Example of what rectal manometry recordings show.

who will take a small amount of tissue from the rectal wall. Depending on the depth of biopsy, different information may be obtained.

Tissue from the mucosa and sub-mucosa can be examined for the presence or absence of ganglia cells only from the superficial nerve plexuses. However, if a full thickness biopsy is taken, it will provide the opportunity to examine for ganglia from both the myenteric and submucous nerve plexuses. Histochemical examination can be carried out on this sample to confirm the absence of ganglial cells (Clayden & Agnarsson 1991).

Ghosh & Griffiths (1998) carried out a retrospective review of rectal biopsies performed on 141 children. They compared the age of onset of the child's symptoms with the diagnosis of Hirschsprung's disease from the biopsy. Their work showed that just 17 of the children who underwent a biopsy had Hirschsprung's disease and all of these had constipation which started in the first 4 weeks of life. While some of the children who were referred for biopsy were older than neonates, all of those diagnosed with Hirschsprung's disease had symptoms starting within this 4-week period. They concluded that if a child's symptoms started after the neonatal period, a biopsy was not necessary.

Box 4.1 Points to remember

- There are many different tests undertaken to help with a diagnosis and for a complete assessment—some routine, some only if indicated.
- Urinalysis is vital to exclude other problems including UTI.
- Some blood tests could become routine; others are for specialist centres or research only.
- X-rays, while useful, must be used carefully and for the purpose of giving as much information as possible, e.g. marker studies rather than plain abdominal X-ray.
- Rectal examinations are rarely used in the UK, except for biopsy under general anaesthetic.
- Skilled paediatric operators should be employed during biopsy taking, and in the histological examination of the tissue.

REFERENCES

Bayer Diagnostics (undated) A practical guide to urine analysis. Bayer, Newbury

Blethyn A J, Jenkins H R, Roberts R, Jones K Verrier 1995a Radiological evidence of constipation in urinary tract infection. Archives of Disease in Childhood 73(6): 534–535

Blethyn A J, Jones K Verrier, Newcombe R, Roberts G M, Jenkins H R 1995b Radiological assessment of constipation. Archives of Disease in Childhood 73(6): 532–533

Clayden G, Agnarsson U 1991 Constipation in childhood. Oxford University Press, Oxford

Getliffe K, Dolman M 1997 Promoting continence: a clinical and research resource. Baillière Tindall, London

Ghosh A, Griffiths D M 1998 Rectal biopsy in the investigation of constipation. Archives of Disease in Childhood 79(3): 266–268

Kamm M A, Lennard-Jones J E (eds) 1994 Constipation. Wrightson Biomedical Publishing, Petersfield

Stern H P, Stroh S E, Fiedorek S C et al 1995 Increased plasma levels of pancreatic polypeptide and decreased plasma levels of motilin in encopretic children. Pediatrics 96(1): 111–117

Management: Stage 1

Once the full assessment and any necessary investigations have been carried out, one must consider the most appropriate management for the individual child's condition. Each child and their family must be assessed and treated as an individual case, and the management programme must be designed around their circumstances. Having said that, there are four main stages to the treatment and management of the condition: education of the parent and child, the evacuation of the bowel, the maintenance and finally the withdrawal of treatment. Education forms a large part of the management and should be included in all stages of treatment. If the child and parent understand why you are suggesting certain things, it is easier for them to comply. This chapter and the following two will look at each of the other stages in turn.

PREPARATION

An important aspect of the management of children with chronic functional constipation with overflow soiling is to dispel any myths or mistaken beliefs and to involve the child as well as the parent/carer in the treatment. Much of the time during the first few appointments with these children and their families should be devoted to explaining the condition and the management as fully as possible. Patients and their families need to be completely clear about the regime which is being designed around their needs in order that compliance or concordance with the programme is achieved. This regime will to some extent dominate their lives for the foreseeable future, so their agreement to follow it is vital. Use of good quality visual aids to fully explain the condition, its possible causes and the aims of its management help understanding. (See Chapter 9 for further information about visual aids that have been found to be effective). The professional must be sure they completely understand what they are talking about; any uncertainty will be detected and the child's confidence in the professional's ability to manage the problem will suffer. This is a distressing condition and, as already discussed, the family may have attempted to get help elsewhere on previous occasions. The family have often been given many different descriptions of the condition. Your knowledge may be good, but if the ability to communicate it to the child and the parents is lacking, this will also have an adverse effect on their confidence in you. Talking to child and parent in language they understand is a vital aspect of the management.

DOCUMENTATION

All discussion concerning stages of the management, choice of laxative and goals to be set for each step of the programme should be done while the child and parent are with the health professional managing the case. These must be documented clearly in the child's records. This helps when the child and parent return for the next appointment, as the plan is written down and can be referred to. Patients should be asked whether they have been carrying out agreed plans. If not, discuss the reason; if there is a genuine problem establish whether this can be overcome or whether the programme needs altering.

There is also an obvious legal and professional need to ensure good comprehensive record keeping with any patient/client in your care. The UKCC (1998) states:

Record keeping is an integral part of nursing, midwifery and health visiting practice. It is a tool of professional practice and one which should help the care process. It is not separate from this process and it is not an optional extra to be fitted in if circumstances allow.

Obviously, if you have access to a purpose-designed tool to record the required information, this is somewhat easier, but whatever the method of record keeping, care plans for each child must be documented. If there is a local decision to use generic notes for recording these appointments, it would be useful to have a printed list of questions that must be asked. This enables the professional to adhere to the same format of assessment with each child. Another benefit of keeping a good record of the child and parent's progress is that, at times when they are losing heart, looking back gives the opportunity to remind them just how much they have already achieved so far. When the child and parent are closely involved with the management for long periods of time, it can be impossible for them to remember their own situation when they first attended. What their own hopes and fears regarding the condition were, and their feelings about the plight they felt themselves to be in become distant memories for them. A few words in your records can help them to acknowledge improvements and celebrate their success thus far.

While a number of clients will have a similar management plan for their condition, is your own memory sufficient to remember why this particular child needed something different? If you are seeing more than a couple of children with this condition, it becomes difficult even for those with extremely efficient memories to recall deviations from the standard treatment plan and why they were put into place at the time. However, when one starts auditing the efficacy of different plans at a later date, this can become impossible. Documenting the reasons for any slight changes can help with this process. Auditing your success rate or dropout rate is a vital component of developing your practice overall, but it is also a major part of the individual child's care plan. Assessing, planning, implementing and evaluating care is a routine we all follow each time a nursing or medical intervention is carried out for our patients.

EXPLANATIONS

In order for both child and parent to be able to participate in their own management plan, they should be given information that allows them to understand what is being asked of them and how it will benefit them. An explanation of the condition at a level that they both understand is the first step in achieving this. As health professionals we are familiar with the term 'constipation' and 'mega rectum' means something to us; this is not so for the general public. The judicious use of language and visual aids can reap rewards far in excess of the effort used in finding the correct way to explain the condition. If the family refer to it as 'poo', then use that word. If they use a word you are less comfortable with, agree between you what is an acceptable word and document it. Whatever visual aids you use must be ones you feel comfortable with. If the thought of clay models of faeces is not to your liking then use the parent or child's verbal description. If you travel to a different location when seeing children with soiling problems, another factor is brought into the choice of visual aids—they must be easily transported and carried. Remember, though, that some anatomical diagrams can be very complex even to health professionals, so for someone with no real knowledge of what the body's organs look like or what tasks they perform, simplicity is the key to aiding understanding. Draw your own or refer to children's books for clear and simple diagrams of the anatomy of the body.

When explaining the reason why this child has a problem, discuss issues raised as honestly as possible and if the answer is not clear then say so. This is a time when familial problems may be discussed; if another member of the family has a less severe problem use this information to aid their understanding. Mother has a problem of constipation and older brother only goes to the toilet twice a week but with no soiling—this child just has the family problem but in a more severe form. This results in his other problem of leaking and if you can explain why that happens too, so that the family can understand, you will have made the first major step in the child's management.

Discuss treatment options not in the abstract but by detailing exactly what they entail and what impact they could have on the family's life. Do they wish the child to be admitted to hospital, if possible or necessary, for the evacuation of the bowel? Do they understand that some methods will take longer than others, but may cause less disruption to the family's routine? Have they tried anything in the past that they feel has failed and do they want to avoid it in the future? Perhaps most important is explaining why the treatment will take as long as you are predicting. One mother attending my clinic told me I was the seventh person she had been to see, including a consultant paediatric surgeon, a homeopath and a clinical psychologist. Her biggest problem was that all clinicians (except the psychologist who, because of a long waiting list, had sent her to me for discussion first) had 'sent her away to do things' and she had not felt able to do them without very regular support, which was missing. Ascertain what the family's expectations of you and your management are. Are they realistic? Can you help them to accept more realistic aims of your treatment plan? If this is not possible, both they and you may have to accept that you are not the right professional to support them through this long and sometimes trying process. Some parents want a quick fix, something which is not possible for this condition. Magic wands are not standard issue for any health professional, much as we would like them at times!

Laxatives

As laxatives play a large part in the management of these children, they and their parents must be clear about the use and action of drugs prescribed. What is a stool softener and what is a stimulant, and why do we use both? What different types of each group of laxative are there; is one more palatable than another (see Chapter 6)? How long will the child have to take them for? What do the parents do if the child refuses to take them? It helps if the health professional has tasted some of the products prescribed or recommended; some are unpleasant, others are more palatable, and others are disgusting.

Diet

Diet plays a role too. What changes do the parents need to make to the family's eating habits? The whole family will undoubtedly benefit from a healthier eating plan, and the child will not feel so isolated if all the family have the same meals. Try to advise on ways of introducing fibre so that it is not too recognisable. Drinking habits for this child, and very likely for the others in the family, need to be examined. More information on this is given in Chapter 6, but the explanation about the importance of these factors must be good enough to encourage them to make the required changes.

Some treatment options may require a written consent from the child, and particularly from the parent, and if the explanations given are adequate they will help to form the informed aspect of the consent obtained. If the explanations are not adequate and the results of the treatment are disappointing to the family, the professional must accept some of the blame. It is very likely that more time spent talking about it could have prevented the feeling of failure.

CHOICE

Once these explanations are complete and both child and parent have the information required, guidance can be given to enable them to make choices about their management plan. As the UKCC (1992) states: 'work in an open and co-operative manner with patients, clients and their families, foster their independence and recognise and respect their involvement in the planning and delivery of care.'

If the family are uncertain whether they can deal with a particular treatment option, look to alternatives and help them to make the right selection from the options available. If the child and his parent have helped to plan their own treatment they are more likely to adhere to it. When treatments do not fit an individual's lifestyle, it makes it less likely the treatment will be complied with. The various treatment options will be discussed more fully below.

TREATMENT OPTIONS FOR EVACUATION OF THE BOWEL

Introduction

Once an individual child's situation has been assessed and the treatment choices have been made, the first stage in the manage-

---

Box 5.1   Points to remember

- Prepare both the child and his family and yourself. Visual aids, notes for documentation; **know** your subject.
- Documentation is vital. Not only is it a legal and professional requirement, it also aids your memory for the next visit.
- Audit your success as well as your clients'.
- Visual aids can help you explain the condition, **but** only if you are comfortable using them.
- Explain what will happen and how it will affect the family, **do not** use abstract descriptions.
- **Try** the things you recommend—laxatives (only a small taste), particular foods, etc.
- Help clients to make an **informed** choice about their own treatment plan.

ment of the condition may be commenced. Many of the children who soil have been constipated for a considerable period of time, and the rectum is almost certainly faecally loaded. The colon may also be loaded and, in order to begin the longer term management of the child's condition, this must be evacuated. Various methods are employed to evacuate the bowel depending upon the degree of faecal loading and the family's ability to deal with each of these.

Stool softeners

The simplest method of evacuating the bowel is to give large doses of a stool softener such as lactulose two or three times a day for 2 to 3 weeks. Of course, this may be very effective if the child is given sufficient doses over a long enough time span. One major problem with this technique is that patients may lose what little control they have over their bowels and the soiling may increase dramatically until the colon is empty. If children and their parents are forewarned of this, and still wish to go ahead, it may be acceptable to them. Bear in mind that, however badly you paint the picture of what may happen, they will not quite believe it and will think you are exaggerating to some extent.

Few children like the taste of lactulose—as society has changed and become aware of healthier options, young children today are given fewer very sweet things to eat, and lactulose is extremely sweet. However, when the other option is methylcellulose, many will choose lactulose. Make suggestions for reducing the sweetness—patients can disguise the taste with juice or cordial, or counteract the sweetness with a squirt of lemon juice. If the child really cannot cope with it, try a different stool softener. Stools can be softened with either an osmotic laxative, a surfactant or a detergent.

Whatever stool softener is chosen, the dose given must be large enough to ensure that the faeces in the colon will be evacuated. For infants under the age of one, softening the retained stool and then changing diet and fluid intake will often cure the condition completely. Some may need an osmotic laxative in the longer term and the use of fibre in the diet as a natural stimulant— prunes or rhubarb, for example.

Clayden (1996) suggests that if this alone is ineffective, the child should move on to a crescendo of methods to evacuate the bowel, while others (Muir 1999) suggest that, after a week of soft-eners, other types of laxative should be added routinely. Clayden's Crescendo:

1. senna (Senokot syrup or senna tablets) in a single daily but incremental dose until stool is passed *but* colic may be caused and soiling increased if stool too hard or too large
2. sodium picosulfate (sodium picosulfate elixir or Picolax sachets) *but* often violent effect
3. polyethylene glycol (KleanPrep or Golytely) *but* large volumes are required and there may be difficulty in drinking the necessary amount, which may be overcome by passage of nasogastric tube, however this may be more stressful than:
4. enema (micro or phosphate enema) *but* this will add to the fear/discomfort and may intensify defecation avoidance and patient's mistrust of medical and nursing staff unless the child fully understands and cooperates with (or administers) it
5. manual evacuation under general anaesthetic *but* this has the risks associated with anaesthesia, although it allows a careful examination for ectopia and stenosis and an anal dilatation, which may be valuable in the situation of massive mega rectum where the smooth muscle of the rectal wall, including the anal sphincter, is hypertrophied. This can also be combined with a rectal biopsy in persisting cases or where the age of the child, age of onset and relative lack of overflow soiling may suggest the possibility of late presentation or previously missed very short segment Hirschsprung's disease.

Stimulant laxatives

As mentioned above, Clayden suggests starting with the most commonly prescribed stimulant laxative, senna, a plant deriva-tive. While this is effective in many cases of fairly acute cases of constipation, for children who have suffered from this condition for prolonged periods and who may have the whole colon load-ed with faeces, senna may cause problems. Senna is a mild stim-ulant, but even so can cause quite severe abdominal cramps during its action. These abdominal cramps can lead to a lack of compliance by patients—is anyone really happy to continue tak-ing any medication they know is going to cause discomfort?

Usually given at night, senna produces a result approximately 6–8 hours later in cases of acute constipation. These children are likely to need very large doses of senna to achieve a result—30 ml daily.

Sodium picosulfate is described in most drug books as a mild stimulant. Any individual who has taken it will tell you this is a vast understatement. The contents of the sachet are mixed with water and an exothermic reaction occurs in the glass (it becomes warm). Taken at any time during the day, it gives a rapid and explosive result within a couple of hours.

Movicol is a new laxative that is not yet licensed for use in children, but some teams are carrying out trials with it and obtaining very favourable results. It has two actions, as it both softens and stimulates the passing of any faecal mass in the bowel. It is classed as an iso-osmotic laxative as it is based upon the polyethylene glycol solutions used for bowel cleansing, however the solution is at a different concentration, which means that there is less risk of electrolyte imbalance after administration.

Bisacodyl can also be used at this stage. This comes in the form of a tablet which cannot be crushed or dissolved, but as it is only the size of the oral contraceptive pill it can be swallowed by many children. Its use can result in severe abdominal pain or explosive diarrhoea.

Polyethylene glycol lavage

Polyethylene glycol is also known as the proprietary brand KleanPrep or Golytely and is used prior to major bowel surgery to ensure the bowel is empty. For this method to be used successfully in these children, they must be admitted to hospital for the duration of the procedure. The child has to be old enough to understand a full explanation of the procedure. He may need sedation to have a nasogastric tube passed and may require an enema prior to the polyethylene glycol. The dose is calculated on the child's body weight and is based on 10–40 ml per kilo and given at a rate of 300 ml per hour via the nasogastric tube. This may continue for 2 to 5 days until the solution, which is pink to begin with, is passed as pink faeces. The child can drink unlimited amounts during the treatment. Some children find it causes vomiting; if this occurs, try slowing the rate at which the fluid is given. It may also cause hypokalaemia, which will require potassium to be given orally. The child undergoing this procedure will require intensive monitoring. The child may be confused by the necessity of having a nasogastric tube passed when the problem is with his bottom. Children have very simplistic views about what happens to them and around them, so explanations have to be prepared carefully; expect some unusual questions from the child.

Enemata

There are two main types of enemata in common use today: the micro enema and the phosphate enema. Different health service units will have policies regarding which type they wish to be used in varying age groups. Some will not permit the use of phosphate enemas for children under 3, or under 5; others will not permit their use in children at all. Ensure your knowledge of local policy is up-to-date. The reason for this unwillingness to use phosphate enemata in children is that it can cause quite devastating electrolyte imbalance.

Micralax enemata do not have this effect, and are therefore safer to use when treating children. Both the BNF and MIMS state that these are suitable only for children over the age of 3 years. They are made up of a sodium citrate solution which acts by osmosis to soften the stool. The size of the dose also makes them more acceptable when treating children: the volume is only 5 ml of fluid to be given per rectum.

Whatever the type of enema to be given, there are some things to consider beforehand. The first factor is the age of the child—Clayden (1996), as already mentioned, suggests it may be appropriate to give intravenous sedation to children prior to the administration of an enema. The sedation may be continued until there has been a result from the enema; some children will have an exceptionally large and potentially painful stool to pass as a result of the enema. He also suggests that the older child may be taught to self-administer the enema. This may take a large amount of patience for the staff supporting the young person through this.

If a member of staff is to administer the enema, all usual local policies and procedures for this should be adhered to. The child should be given a full explanation, including details of the possible result, and the child's dignity and privacy should be respected while the procedure takes place. The child has to lie on their left side and the staff member should be wearing gloves and have all the necessary equipment to hand. The tube to be inserted should be lubricated and inserted slowly and carefully into the anus and via the anal canal to the lower section of the rectum to the required depth. The contents of the enema are then expelled by squeezing the container. While keeping the container closed, it should be withdrawn and disposed of in the usual manner as clinical waste.

Easy and swift access to a toilet, with some privacy, is the next desirable requirement for anyone who has had an enema. While the phosphate enema is rapid-acting, the Micralax will have a result in approximately 20 minutes.

While they are, on occasion, the method of choice to evacuate the faecally loaded bowel, enemata are not pleasant procedures for anyone to undergo. To a child with limited understanding of the procedure, they can be a major trial, and our job as health professionals is to ensure the child is as prepared as possible to deal with the situation. As discussed earlier in the text, sexual abuse can be a cause of soiling, so any treatment which is carried out around the anogenital area should be considered very carefully before it is chosen. This possibility is one of the reasons why it may be advisable for the older child with sufficient understanding to self-administer the enema. Anything which has any sexual connotations should be avoided, if at all possible. If this is not possible, the child should be involved as much as possible, either by self-administering or by choosing the person who should administer the enema. At times, a parent may be the chosen person to administer the enema and they will therefore require careful teaching on the technique.

Manual evacuation

It is to be hoped that few, if any, children will have to undergo a manual evacuation of faeces under general anaesthetic. Some will, however, because other methods fail or because the assessment and investigations show that the degree of faecal loading is so great that all the other methods would result in problems. Buchanan (1992) recounts the findings on abdominal X-ray of a child who had had a barium enema 3 months prior to the marker studies for which the X-ray had been performed. The X-ray quite clearly showed a very large faecal mass, almost the size of the pelvic outlet, outlined in the barium medium given 3 months earlier, as well as the radioopaque markers given for this investigation.

A faecal mass of this magnitude would be extremely difficult to pass and would cause severe pain, so a manual evacuation would be the only appropriate method to empty the bowel. As a large part of the management of chronic constipation and soiling is to avoid recurrences of pain on defecation, this is a sensible option in this type of case.

The parents will require a full explanation in order for you to secure informed written consent for the procedure to be carried out. The child obviously has to be given a general anaesthetic to allow this procedure to be carried out. It must be ascertained that the child does not have any other pre-existing condition that will impact on the general anaesthesia. Any general anaesthetic carries with it a risk of problems, but in most cases this is minimal. Once the child is anaesthetised, the surgeon can begin to remove the faecal mass in small pieces. With very severely impacted faeces, this can take a little time. At the completion of this task, the surgeon has the opportunity to perform an anal dilatation if this is indicated, or to take a biopsy if this is felt to be necessary. As discussed in the previous chapter, there is a school of thought that suggests this may only be necessary if the child's symptoms started within 4 weeks of birth, but others feel that short or ultra-short segment Hirschsprung's disease may not manifest until later. The individual surgeon will, therefore, have his own ideas concerning the necessity of a biopsy. It is also to be remembered that other neurogenic conditions may be discovered during the examination of the tissue. If it is short segment Hirschsprung's disease, there is no guarantee that the correct length of colon will be selected from which to take the biopsy. Biopsy may be taken by suction, which removes tissue from the mucosa and sub-mucosa, or it may be necessary to take a full-thickness biopsy to ensure a wide range of investigations can be performed on the tissue (see Chapter 4).

Anal dilatation can help when the rectum is excessively large and requires a large volume of faeces to stimulate the defecation reflex. Dilatation results in reduced activity of the anal sphincter and means a reduced rectal volume is required before the pressure rises to the level needed to allow defecation. In babies and young children one little finger, well lubricated, inserted gently into the anus and left there for a few minutes can be successful. It often needs repeating. For older children this should be performed under a general anaesthetic, so a manual evacuation offers an ideal opportunity to carry out this procedure too. Clayden & Agnarsson (1991) suggest: 'The anus is gently stretched by both index fingers until both middle fingers can be inserted as well. The stretch should not be forced and should last several minutes.'

SUMMARY

Each child is an individual, and management should, to some extent, be individually tailored. To help this, both child and parents should be guided towards the appropriate management plan. This will be achieved if they are given full explanations at a level commensurate with their level of understanding. All decisions taken should be documented in the relevant records.

The first stage of management is to empty the bowel of any faecal mass which has accumulated there. There are a number of methods that may be employed for this:

- Stool softeners in larger than usual doses for 2 to 3 weeks, which may have the desired effect but may cause a worsening of the symptoms for a while
- Stimulant laxatives may be added; these might cause abdominal pain but may not clear a bowel that shows white out on the X-ray
- KleanPrep needs hospital admission but is very effective
- Enemata are unpleasant and only empty the lower rectum, so again a white out on X-ray may not be cleared

---

BOX 5.2   Points to remember

The choice of method employed to evacuate the bowel will depend upon:
- Severity of the faecal loading
- Child's and parent's choice
- The need to carry out other investigations or procedures
- Past history
- The time frame
- Choice can be helped by ensuring that the child and parent understand **all** the options available to them
- Informed consent will be required for some of the methods—ensure it **is** informed

- Manual evacuation carries the risks associated with general anaesthetic but can enable both rectal biopsy and anal dilatation to be carried out at the same time.

REFERENCES

Buchanan 1992 Children who soil, assessment and treatment. John Wiley, Chichester
Clayden G, Agnarsson U 1991 Constipation in childhood. Oxford University Press, Oxford
Clayden G 1996 A guide for good practice: childhood constipation. Ambulatory Child Health 1(5): 250–255
Muir J 1999 Guidelines for the management of childhood constipation. Reckitt & Colman Products, Hull
UKCC 1992 Code of professional conduct. UKCC, London
UKCC 1998 Guidelines for records and record keeping. UKCC, London

6

Management: Stage 2

INTRODUCTION

Once the bowel has been emptied, by whatever method, the management of the chronic constipation can move on to the next stage. This next stage is referred to as maintenance: it is the time when the child takes laxatives regularly and these, together with the diet and fluid intake, are adjusted until at least one daily bowel movement is occurring. Choice of laxatives and therapy combination depends on professional preference or local policy. What dietary advice is given may be influenced by the ease of access to a dietician locally. If a dietician is not readily available, the nursing and medical staff must take on the role of giving appropriate dietary advice. During this stage of treatment a high level of support is needed for both child and parents, although less support is needed as they progress on the programme. The whole family are likely to have questions and comments on the management plan and they need access to the professional supporting them in order to clarify these points. The child will probably be withdrawn and almost always miserable before starting a management plan, for a number of reasons. First, due to the very physical effects of constipation; second, because of the teasing they have endured and third, due to the fact that past efforts at clearing the problem have often failed—sometimes because of lack of support. The changes that take place in the child's personality as bowel control is regained can be dramatic and extremely pleasing to both the family and the health professional managing their care.

The management plan should have the overall aim of solving the child's constipation and soiling problems, but it may have smaller objectives along the way, including establishing a routine for the child and changing the diet of the family.

Clayden & Agnarsson (1991) suggest:

The basic plan should be to:

- explain the problem fully
- use the minimum therapeutic input
- ensure complete evacuation of retained stools
- maintain regularity of bowel movements
- establish effective toiletting routines
- monitor progress (charts, consultations—personal and telephone)
- support child and family through the difficult times
- establish information network to ensure the above management.

Some aspects of this management plan have already been discussed in detail; others will be described in the pages that follow.

LAXATIVES

One of the first parts of the plan to be established is what laxatives are to be taken. As already mentioned, there are different types of laxative with different roles in the treatment of constipation. The British National Formulary (BNF) divides laxatives into five groups; bulk-forming laxatives, faecal softeners, osmotic laxatives, stimulant laxatives, and bowel-cleansing solutions. Table 6.1 splits laxatives into these groups, and gives doses and some proprietary names of these preparations. A more detailed discussion on the mode of action and ease of use or acceptability follows.

Box 6.1 Points to remember

- All management issues should be considered together
- Frequent appointments are required in the early stages of management
- Look at the whole family's diet, not just that of the child being treated
- Involve the family as much as possible in decisions

Table 6.1 Laxatives, type and dose

Type	Active ingredient	Proprietary names	Dose
Bulk-forming	Ispaghula husk	Fybogel Isogel Regulan Konsyl	Child 6–12 years: $1/_2$-1 level 5 ml spoon. Not recommended for children under 6 years
	Methylcellulose	Celevac	3–6 tablets twice daily with at least 300 ml water
Faecal softeners	Liquid paraffin	Liquid paraffin Oral emulsion	Children over 3 years of age only. 10–40 ml at night
	Docusate sodium	Dioctyl Docusol (Norgalax—enema, not for children)	6 months–2 years: 12.5 mg t.d.s.; over 2 years: 12.5–25 mg t.d.s.
		Fletcher's enemette	Under 3 years: not recommended. Over 3 years: as adult.
Osmotic laxatives	Magnesium and sodium salts	Epsom salts, Andrews liver salts. Magnesium hydroxide	As label; not usually recommended for children
	Phosphates	Phosphate enema	Over 3 years: dose according to body weight
	Sodium citrate	Micolette, Micralax and Relaxit Micro-enema	Child over 3 years: 5–10 ml (as adult)
	Disaccharide	Lactulose, Duphalac	Children < 1 year: 2.5 ml b.d., 1–4 years: 5 ml b.d.; 5–10 years: 10 ml b.d.; adults 15 ml b.d. or more
		Lactugal	Not for children < 1 year, otherwise as above
		Lactitol	Children 1–6 years: 1/4–1/2 sachet daily, 6–12 years: 1/2–1 sachet daily; 12–16 years: 1–2 sachets daily

Table 6.1 (Contd.)

Type	Active ingredient	Proprietary names	Dose
Iso-osmotic laxatives	Polyethylene glycol, sodium bicarbonate, sodium chloride and potassium chloride	Movicol	Sachets that are reconstituted in water—at present not recommended for use in children, although some centres are carrying out clinical trials and getting good results
		KleanPrep	Not recommended in MIMS but used in some centres: 10–40 ml per kilo body weight, 300 ml/h via nasogastric tube
Stimulant laxatives	Senna	Senokot tablets, granules and syrup	Under 2 years: not recommended; 2–6 years: 2.5–5 ml; over 6 years: 5–10 ml daily
	Sodium picosulfate	Sodium picosulfate liquid, Laxoberal liquid,	0–5 years: 2.5 ml; 5–10 years 2.5–5 ml; > 10 years 5–15 ml nocte
		Picolax	1–2 years: 1/4 sachet; 2–4 years: 1/2 sachet; 4–9 years: 1 sachet daily; > 9 years: 1 + sachet, as required for result
	Bisacodyl	Bisacodyl 5 mg tabs or suppositories 5 mg and 10 mg Dulcolax 5 mg tabs and suppositories 5 mg and 10 mg	Children under 10 years: 1 tab nocte or 1 × 5 mg suppository, morning; over 10: as adult, 10 mg tablet or 10 mg suppository
Bowel-cleansing solutions	Sodium Picosulfate	Sodium picosulfate and picolax	As before
	Polyethylene glycol	KleanPrep	As before

Bulk-forming laxatives

Often derived from either methylcellulose or ispaghula husk, these are useful for forming a larger volume of stool. They should be used only when increasing dietary fibre is unsuccessful or contraindicated because of other conditions. Another aspect of taking any bulking laxative is the need to remind the child of increased fluid intake required when using these preparations. As they retain water in the contents of the colon, they are effective in softening the stool, as well as adding bulk, making them easier to pass. This is obviously important in children who have experienced painful bowel movements in the past.

A natural bulk-forming dietary additive is unprocessed wheat bran; this may be added to other foods, for example soups, to provide fibre. It is not the most palatable of substances, however, and should be avoided if at all possible. Larger fluid intake volumes are required with this, as it is dry.

Faecal softeners

These act as a lubricant to the stool. Such laxatives are therefore particularly useful if there has been anal pain due to fissure or haemorrhoids. (There are also laxatives in other groups which have softening properties, including docusate sodium which, because of its detergent action, reduces surface tension and may increase absorption of other drugs.) The most well known faecal softener is liquid paraffin. It is not used often in children, and the Committee on Safety of Medicines (CSM) has recommended avoiding prolonged use and has stated that it is contraindicated for those under 3 years of age. Problems with liquid paraffin use are rare, although it may be aspirated and cause lipid pneumonia. This potential problem obviously precludes it being given to anyone with swallowing problems.

Another potential problem is that the liquid paraffin may seep out of the anus, causing skin irritation. Finally, liquid paraffin may interfere with absorption of some fat-soluble vitamins. All these side-effects support the recommendation that it should not be used for prolonged periods of time. Mineral oils such as liquid paraffin are used far more routinely in the USA as a first line treatment for chronic constipation.

Osmotic laxatives

As suggested by the name, these work by osmosis, keeping fluid within the stool which makes it softer and therefore easier to pass. They can be administered orally or per rectum. There are two main types of osmotic laxatives: the saline purgatives and the disaccharide solution. Saline purgatives include magnesium salts (Epsom salts), magnesium hydroxide (Milk of Magnesia-type medications) and phosphate enemata, as well as sodium salts. Because of the risk of sodium and water retention as a result of too much sodium in susceptible individuals, these should be avoided. Hypernatraemia is potentially fatal in young infants and therefore these should never be used in the very young. There is evidence that magnesium salts promote the release of cholecystokinin, which increases intestinal motility. Other members of this group are sodium picosulfate and polyethylene glycol, which will be covered in more detail in other sections. The disaccharide group includes lactulose, a semi-synthetic substance which is not absorbed from the gastrointestinal tract and therefore remains in the contents until reaching the colon, where it provides food for the lactobacilli there. This results in a higher bacterial content of the stool and an increased amount of lactic acid and formic acid, which provide the molecules which cause the osmosis and water retention in the stool.

Lactulose is usually better tolerated by children than the bulk-forming methylcellulose. Glycerine suppositories also fall within this group of medications, although they probably have some stimulant action because of the irritant property of glycerol. Administered per rectum, they act to draw water into the stool and therefore soften it. The Micralax enema mentioned in the previous chapter is also a member of this group. Sodium citrate, sodium alkylsulphoacetate, sorbic acid, and glycerol and sorbitol mixed give ample opportunity for osmosis to occur.

Stimulant laxatives

These act on the intestines and increase the motility of the colon, but as a result can cause colicky pain about which the child and parent should be warned. These laxatives are helpful, however, because they can be used to time visits to the toilet. Obviously, they must be avoided in intestinal obstruction and should not be used until any faecal evacuation has been completed or the faecal mass has been softened sufficiently. Common members of this group are senna, sodium picosulfate, bisacodyl and danthron. Although most are administered orally, there is a bisacodyl suppository which may be given. Prolonged use in adults is not advised because of the risk of abuse and the chance of developing an atonic colon. As Clayden & Agnarsson (1991) report, 'They are all subject to laxative abuse in adults and may cause toxic degeneration of myenteric plexuses and hence interference with colonic motility.'

Senna is the most commonly used stimulant laxative as its action is fairly predictable and it produces fewer side-effects than others. It reaches the large bowel between 6 to 24 hours after ingestion and its action can therefore be anticipated around this time, although in children it is usually nearer 12 to 24 hours after taking it.

Sodium picosulfate is a very strong stimulant laxative and therefore gives very painful abdominal cramps which can lead to lack of concordance, with children refusing to take it. Clayden & Agnarsson (1991) suggest there are frequently made mistakes when using senna which can also be applied to the use of any stimulant laxative. These are:

- Using senna before complete evacuation of old, retained stools leads to abdominal colic and an increase in overflow soiling
- Used too frequently and ignoring the time lapse from ingestion to action (usually 12–24 hours in children). A daily or alternate day dose is to be preferred to any other regime
- Using senna for too short a time, giving insufficient opportunity for the bowel habit to become established and the child's confidence to consolidate
- Not warning children and parents that a year or more on senna may be necessary
- Not using methyl cellulose or lactulose to maintain a soft but bulky stool.

I think I would also add: incorrect dose being prescribed—either too much or too little. Too much will result in more severe abdominal cramps, which neither the child nor parent wishes to endure, and too little is obviously not effective.

Certain foodstuffs have actions very like the stimulant laxatives, including rhubarb, prunes and liquorice. These can be safely used in young children to maintain an appropriately regular bowel evacuation, without the need to give laxatives.

Bowel-cleansing solutions

These solutions are particularly intended to clean the gut prior to intestinal surgery or radiological examination of the intestine, and are not an accepted treatment for constipation per se. However, the nature of the condition being discussed is not ordinary constipation, and in extraordinary circumstances, special treatments are adopted. In these cases two of the bowel-cleansing solutions are used: KleanPrep and sodium picosulfate; although the latter is, strictly speaking, a stimulant laxative, it has been adopted for this use. While the KleanPrep is used as the primary evacuator of the bowel, some children may be prescribed sodium picosulfate as the stimulant laxative of choice or as an adjunct to another such as senna. The child takes senna daily but adds in a dose of picosulfate at weekends if there has not been a stool for an agreed length of time.

Laxative regimes

For the management of this condition to be effective, it is essential that the laxatives be used in the correct order and in the right combination. Stimulants alone are insufficient as they will result in the child passing perhaps a small hard painful stool. Softeners, too, will be ineffective when used alone, as they will soften the stool but the volume of the faeces will continue to build up in the rectum and be passed infrequently.

As it is not desirable for the child to rely on laxatives for life, it is vital that we also attempt to make changes to the other common causes of constipation such as poor diet and inadequate fluid intake. To be successful, all aspects of the management of constipation must be considered together. In Chapter 5, we considered the evacuation of the bowel and looked at the methods to be employed for this; we have now examined the different types of laxatives and their appropriate use. The combination of two laxatives can be the making of the management plan for each individual child.

First, a laxative that will soften the stool has to be selected; the commonest in use is lactulose. For those children who do not like its taste, other options may be Fybogel, a bulking agent, or docusate sodium, a faecal softener—whichever the child finds more palatable. The dose may need adjustment to suit individual children to maintain soft, but not loose, stools which are easy to pass. These laxatives are usually given twice daily, morning and night. While these will give volume and softness to the stool, they will not in most cases give the urge to defecate. To encourage regular bowel movements, a stimulant laxative must be added. Again, finding the correct one for each individual needs some time investment, but the result should be worthwhile. Once the correct type of stimulant is chosen, the dose may need adjustment so that the child is passing one soft stool daily. Although they are usually given at night, the time of administration may need some variation so that the stool is passed at a convenient time for the child and his family. If last thing at night produces a result at 10 a.m. the next day, this may be inconvenient because it is school time or playgroup time. In this case, the dose must be taken earlier in the day. If the child is woken early in the morning to the call to stool, the dose time needs to be later. The dose of the laxative needs adjusting too, if there is a problem with abdominal cramps. While some abdominal symptoms are required by some children to make them aware of the need to defecate, too much pain will cause reluctance to continue with the medication. Minor adjustments may solve the problem, or another stimulant altogether may be required. These are common-sense issues, but families often feel the need to be 'given permission' by the health professional to make adjustments. As these are the minor problems that often arise at the start of any treatment plan, it is vital that the child and family have easy, frequent access to the health professional managing the case. This contact may be face to face, or may be by telephone if a query arises between appointments. This

---

Box 6.2   Points to remember

- There are five different groups of laxatives—bulk-forming laxatives
  faecal softeners
  osmotic laxatives
  stimulant laxatives
  bowel-cleansing solutions
- Each has to be used in the correct way and combinations must be used in the right order
- Doses may need adjusting until the optimum is reached and the child has one bowel movement daily
- The family and anyone else involved will have to understand that they will need these medicines for a long period of time
- Regular checks at appointments are vital to help improve concordance

contact can be the one thing that makes the difference between the success or failure of the management plan.

When the laxative regime is settled, it is time for the other aspects of treatment to be tackled. These issues will be detailed over the next pages.

DIET
Introduction

We are all aware that diet plays an important role in maintaining good bowel health; a healthy diet ensures the regular evacuation of the bowel and contributes to a large proportion of the faecal matter passed. For many people, the pattern of bowel evacuations varies little, except when there is a major change of diet or during illness, even if their fibre intake is at times poor. Look at your own fibre intake over the last day or two using Table 6.2. Has your own consumption been at the recommended levels? Were these representative days or were they exceptional? Many individuals will not reach the recommended fibre intake levels, and as health professionals we are perhaps more knowledgeable than the general population and recognise the benefits of fibre in our diet and how to ensure we are eating higher fibre foods. If, as health professionals, even we are failing to eat the recommended levels, think how difficult it must be for those without our knowledge. For the children we are managing, diet can play an important role in the treatment, and we have a duty to impart knowledge to both child and parents on how and why they should achieve the intake recommended.

Importance of a balanced diet

As health professionals, there is a responsibility placed upon nurses and doctors to promote good health. One of the aspects of good health we should be promoting is a healthy, balanced diet. A balanced diet should have foodstuffs from each of the major food groups: protein, carbohydrates, fats, fruit and vegetables and dairy products. By consuming food from each of these groups in different proportions, humans should have all the nutrients required by the body to maintain itself in a state of optimum health. Change that balance and things can fairly rapidly start to fail. Too much fat

Table 6.2   Fibre content of Foods

Food	Amount	Fibre content
Apple	1 average	2.3 g
All Bran	40 g	12 g
Apricots—dried	50 g	12.0 g
Apricots—stewed	50 g	5.0 g
Almonds	25 g	4.1 g
Banana	1 average	3.0 g
Baked beans	225 g	16.4 g
Butter beans	50 g raw wt.	10.8 g
Bran Flakes	25 g	4.3 g
Brussels sprouts	100 g	2.9 g
Broccoli	100 g	4.1 g
Brazil nuts	25 g	3.3 g
Bran Buds	25 g	7.4 g
Brown rice	50 g	2.0 g
Bread—brown	2 slices	3.9 g
Bread—white	25 g	0.8 g
Bread—wholemeal	25 g	2.4 g
Bread—wheatgerm	25 g	1.3 g
Bread—malted	25 g	1.4 g
Bread—hi-bran	25 g	3.1 g
Baked potato	200 g	5.0 g
Beansprouts	25 g	0.3 g
Beetroot	25 g	0.9 g
Blackberries	100 g	7.3 g
Chick peas	50 g raw wt.	7.5 g
Carrots	100 g	3.1 g
Cabbage	100 g	2.8 g
Cornflakes	25 g	3.0 g
Cream crackers	25 g	0.8 g
Crispbread—rye	25 g	3.3 g
Crispbread—wheat	25 g	1.4 g
Celery	25 g	0.5 g
Cucumber	25 g	0.1 g
Cauliflower—boiled	25 g	0.5 g
Courgettes—boiled	25 g	0.3 g
Chips	25 g	0.6 g
Crisps	25 g	1.4–3.2 g
Cranberries	25 g	1.2 g
Chestnuts	25 g	1.9 g
Coconut	25 g	3.8 g
Dates—dried	50 g	4.4 g
Digestive biscuit	25 g	1.5 g
Figs—dried	50 g	9.3 g
Grapes—black	25 g	0.1 g
Grapes—green	25 g	0.3 g
Grapefruit	25 g	0.1 g
Green beans	100 g	3.4 g
Grape nuts	25 g	2.0 g
Hazelnuts	25 g	1.7 g
Kidney beans	50 g raw wt.	12.5 g

Table 6.2 (Contd.)

Food	Amount	Fibre content
Lentils	50 g raw wt.	5.9 g
Lettuce	25 g	0.1 g
Leeks	25 g	1.1 g
Muesli	40 g	4.4 g
Mushrooms	25 g	0.7 g
Marrow	25 g	0.2 g
Melon	25 g	0.3 g
Marmalade	25 g	0.2 g
Mincemeat	25 g	0.9 g
Orange	1 average	3.2 g
Onions—raw	25 g	0.4 g
Onions—spring	25 g	0.9 g
Peas	75 g	9.0 g
Prunes	50 g	8.1 g
Passion fruit	1 average	4.0 g
Pear	1 average	2.6 g
Peanuts	25 g	2.0 g
Pasta—wholemeal	25 g	0.9 g
Peppers	25 g	0.3 g
Porridge oats	50 g	3.4 g
Parsley	25 g	2.5 g
Parsnips	25 g	0.7 g
Potatoes—boiled	25 g	0.3 g
—roasted	25 g	0.6 g
—baked, in skin	25 g	0.7 g
—instant mashed	25 g	1.0 g
Peach	25 g	0.3 g
Plum	25 g	0.6 g
Peanut butter	25 g	2.1 g
Piccalilli	25 g	0.5 g
Pickle, sweet	25 g	0.5 g
Raspberries	100 g	7.4 g
Runner beans	100 g	3.4 g
Rice—white	25 g	0.2 g
Ready Brek	25 g	2.2 g
Rice Krispies	25 g	0.3 g
Radishes	25 g	0.3 g
Redcurrants	25 g	2.3 g
Raisins (sultanas etc.)	25 g	2.0 g
Sweetcorn	100 g	5.7 g
Strawberries	25 g	0.6 g
Split peas	25 g	1.4 g
Shredded Wheat	1 biscuit	2.4 g
Shreddies	25 g	2.3 g
Special K	25 g	0.5 g
Sugar Puffs	25 g	1.7 g
Sultana Bran	25 g	3.6 g
Spaghetti in tomato sauce	25 g	0.3 g
Tomatoes	25 g	0.4 g
Weetabix	1 biscuit	2.2 g
Watercress	25 g	0.9 g

consumed results in weight gain and, in the long term, in obesity. Too few dairy products lowers the calcium intake and can eventually result in osteoporosis. More relevant to this text, too little fibre results in delay in passing stools—constipation. Buchanan (1992) tells us, 'A diet high in protein and/or fats also tends to produce hard constipated stools which are difficult to pass.'

Milk

While lack of fibre is the obvious culprit to consider when looking at the diet of individuals with constipation, there are others that play a role in promoting or preventing good bowel health. Too much or too little of other foods and drinks can impact on the stools formed or the urge to eat fibre-rich foods. Milk is a prime example; while children need a good supply of calcium, most commonly obtained from dairy products, it can fill them up so that they do not wish to eat other foodstuffs that may contain fibre. Iacono et al. (1995), in a small study, found that cow's milk protein could cause an allergic reaction which resulted in chronic constipation. They gave 27 children, aged under 3 years and suffering idiopathic constipation, a cow's milk protein-free diet for a month, then challenged them with cow's milk protein again, and repeated the cycle once more. While on the cow's milk protein-free diet, 21 of the children had a marked improvement in their symptoms, that is they passed more frequent, softer stools and had fewer abdominal symptoms and any anal fissure resolved. When they were challenged with cow's milk protein in their diet, constipation returned within 48–72 hours. They further examined circulating blood levels of Ig E and found that these levels were raised in the children who had an improvement in symptoms while on the cow's milk-free diet. Buchanan (1992) cites work by Davidson et al in 1963 who 'highlighted the role of milk as a causal factor in a soiling problem. It was thought that ingestion of large quantities of milk reduced the desire for other foods, which contain more roughage.'

This knowledge can cause problems when applied to infants who are solely on milk feeds but suffer constipation and abdominal symptoms. The options available to parents have previously been limited to swapping to soya-based formulas; however, these have similar effects to cow's milk and the benefit is therefore questionable. Cow & Gate last year launched a new baby milk formula called Omneo Comfort about which they state: 'This innovative new product may help the large number of parents who come to you with concerns about colic, hard stools, constipation, possetting, etc. without them resorting to medicinal type products' (Cow & Gate, 2000). The formula is apparently totally whey-based and its modified formula features:

- Partially hydrolysed whey protein
- Unique carbohydrate blend: reduced lactose, starch, prebiotic oligosaccharides
- Unique vegetable fat blend: structured vegetable oil
- Vitamins and minerals.

It is not available on prescription but is available in pharmacies and supermarkets. Prebiotics are a recent discovery which appear to be getting good results anecdotally for all sorts of digestive problems, particularly constipation. Foodstuffs including yoghurts and drinks containing a high level of prebiotics are now available at supermarkets.

Fibre

Trying to assess how much fibre a child should eat can be difficult because of the way guidelines in this country are couched. Ask a dietician how much fibre is recommended for a child or an adult, and they will often give it in terms of a percentage of the total daily intake. For a health professional, this can be almost impossible to work out, but for the average family it is a mind-boggling task. The only other guideline is the all-encompassing five portions a day of fruit and vegetables, which would also include other high-fibre foods. The average adult should have 20–30 g of fibre daily, but many do not consume this amount. In the USA when looking at children's diets they use a system of age plus 5, which is much easier. So a 5-year-old child has 5 (years) + 5 = 10 g fibre daily and so on. This makes the task much easier for all concerned and, because it varies with the age of the child, it allows the health professional and the family to know exactly where they stand and how much they have to alter. Giving advice to change the diet to a high-fibre or fibre-rich diet is not sufficient; explicit instructions must be given. McClung et al (1995) found that although families with children with chronic constipation had been told to eat a high-fibre diet, they had not been given enough information on how to do this. When they compared food diaries (or diet logs, as they referred to them), of these families with those of health-conscious families, they found the children with constipation were consuming only one quarter of the fibre recommended. Even the health-conscious, although having good levels of iron, calcium, fat and salt, were only consuming half the recommended amount of fibre. McClung et al (1993) had previously investigated whether a high-fibre diet and laxatives with mineral oil would be safe for children with 'encopresis' to follow and would not result in malnutrition of some degree. They found that, on the contrary, these children suffered no ill effects from following a high-fibre diet in conjunction with the laxative regime, and in fact their constipation symptoms were vastly improved.

Children who have demonstrated a slow transit time should be encouraged to get their fibre intake from fruit and vegetables and should avoid wholegrain fibre. Chiarelli & Markwell (1992) suggest that for those with slow transit, the following foodstuffs should be avoided: wholemeal and wholegrain bread, muesli, bran, cabbage, brussels sprouts, broccoli stalks, dried fruit and nuts. The reason for these recommendations is that because the contents of the bowel are moved along more slowly, there is a greater time for the bacteria to act on it and create greater volumes of gas, which can lead to bloating and abdominal discomfort or pain. The prolonged time in the colon results in more water being absorbed from the contents, making them harder and more painful to pass.

It can be seen that advising on diet can be very complex and it would certainly help to have a table of foodstuffs and their fibre value to give to clients. If you have a good leaflet, it should be used as a stopgap. Table 6.2 can be used to help children and their families.

Making changes to the diet

If there is a dietician available locally for these families, it can only be to their benefit to have expert advice on the changes to be made to their diet. The changes should be recommended for the whole family, and not just the child with symptoms. This avoids further isolation of the patient, and also helps to make the management of the case as simple as possible for the parent. Cooking one meal for the child with the problem and another for the rest of the family leads to complications and possibly to reduced compliance with the programme.

Food diary

To assess any diet, it is important to have a diary of food intake. The length of time the information is collected for may vary, but a minimum of 4 days should give an idea of what the family diet is like. It would be preferable to have a whole week's record of food and drink intake in order to get a more complete picture.

There are many examples of food diaries, and use of locally produced forms is recommended. The information acquired from these can vary from basic to very complex. In the case of the children being treated here, the information required is reasonably basic. There is a need to know what they are eating, in what quantities and at what times during the day. The fluids they drink must also be recorded—again the type and quantity are particularly useful. The example given in Figure 6.1 should cover the basic information required in these cases. This type of food diary, while collecting the information required, is simple in layout and is therefore more 'user-friendly' than some that collect very detailed information. The simplicity results in an increased chance of the family completing the diary as requested. The more complex a form is, the more chance there is of the parent not completing it, either because the task is too daunting or because they do not understand what is required of them.

Box 6.3   Points to remember

- Look at the whole family's eating habits
- Too much or too little of any of the food groups can cause ill effects on the health of an individual
- Milk can cause problems on two counts:
   First, it can cause a child to feel satisfied and not want to eat any higher-fibre foods
   Second, there may be an allergic reaction to cow's milk protein, causing the constipation
- Use of USA system of age +5 g fibre daily is simple to work out and understand
- Good leaflets or food lists with fibre content are useful

FLUID INTAKE

The volume of fluid consumed by children with constipation is vital information. Other information is required too, including the type of fluids they are drinking. Some fluids seem to be better than others at helping to prevent constipation. The role of milk

	Mon.	Tues.	Wed.	Thur.	Fri.	Sat.	Sun.
Breakfast							
Drink							
Mid-a.m.							
Drink							
Lunch							
Drink							
Mid-p.m.							
Drink							
After school							
Drink							
Evening meal							
Drink							
Supper							
Drink							
Snacks							
Drink							

Figure 6.1   Example of a food diary.

Box 6.4 Points to remember

- Use a food diary to collect information on dietary intake—memories are just not accurate enough
- Keep the food diary as simple as possible to ensure it is completed accurately
- Explain how you want it completed—prevent misunderstandings
- Use the information to give advice on dietary changes to be made by the family

---

has already been discussed in the previous section, but larger volumes of tea and coffee seem to have an impact. Chiarelli & Markwell (1992) tell us: 'They also tend to drink less fluid overall, but drink more tea and coffee than others.' This may be due to the caffeine in these drinks having a diuretic effect which impacts on the stool, resulting in it being drier and harder.

Carbonated drinks may cause problems of abdominal discomfort, if the gas they contain builds up in the intestines and becomes trapped, causing a bloated feeling. It is well known that to improve renal health and bowel health, fluid intake must be at the correct volume, but what is the correct volume? Table 3.1 details what volumes children should be drinking on a daily basis to maintain health.

Asking children to increase the volumes they are drinking each day can be problematic. If the child attends school, it may be that only water is provided for them to drink during the school day. Many children today are not used to drinking plain water. Some schools do have peculiar-tasting water. Add all these situations together and it can be seen that increasing the fluid intake may become an insurmountable problem for some children. Many schools are reasonable when approached by parents to explain the rationale behind the request that they be allowed to bring in drinks. Some, however, will remain adamant that the child will have to drink the water provided. Local experience has shown that both these scenarios are possible; sometimes if a health professional explains to teachers that children should drink a certain volume during the day, and if they cannot or will not drink during the long hours they are in school, it could be deleterious to the children's health, this may sway the school's opinion. If it is also explained that children who are dehydrated do not concentrate as well as those who are well hydrated, this too may add to the argument successfully. On my caseload, I saw a young lady with both constipation and wetting problems who had restricted her fluid intake to just a few sips each day. Obviously, she would have been reluctant to increase her fluid intake drastically, so small increases were suggested. She went from five sips at each drink, to ten, then to one quarter of a cup, then half a cup, until she could drink a whole cup several times daily. After increasing to ten sips three or four times daily, she attended another appointment with her mother, who was so impressed with the changes in her daughter. The child was now able to play with other children, where before she did not seem to have the energy to play, and she was improving academically as she could now concentrate for longer periods of time. Mother in fact reported her whole life had changed just by a small increase in fluid intake. She became even better as time went on and she increased her fluid intake further. ERIC (Enuresis Resource and Information Centre) has recently launched a campaign to encourage children to have water to drink in school, and to encourage schools to allow this. The prime reason for this is that it helps the enuretic child to reduce his incidence of wetting. It is to be hoped that this campaign is successful for children with constipation too.

Box 6.5   Points to remember

- Fluid intake plays an important role in general health as well as in bowel health
- Look at recommended levels of fluid intake for body weight and use this for giving advice
- Children will change in other ways once their fluid intake is increased in line with recommended levels
- Use health knowledge to form the argument for drinks to be allowed in school where there are difficulties
- Adequate fluid intake aids concentration—a winner for school staff!

REFERENCES

British Medical Association & Royal Pharmaceutical Society of Great Britain 2000 The British National Formulary Number 40. Pharmaceutical Press, Wallingford
Buchanan A 1992 Children who soil, assessment and treatment. John Wiley, Chichester

Clayden G, Agnarsson U 1991 Constipation in Childhood. Oxford University Press, Oxford

Chiarelli P, Markwell S 1992 Let's get things moving, overcoming constipation. Gore & Osment Publications, Woollahra, NSW

Cow & Gate 2000 A new infant milk for a comfortable digestion and settled bottle-fed babies—advance information. In Practice. Cow & Gate, Sherbourne

Iacono G, Carroccio A, Cavataio F, Montalto G, Cantarero M D, Notarbartolo A, 1995 Chronic constipation as a symptom of cow milk allergy. The Journal of Pediatrics 126(1): 34–39

McClung H J, Boyne L J, Linsheild T, Heitlinger L A, Murray R D, Fyda J, Li B U K 1993 Is combination therapy for encopresis nutritionally safe? Pediatrics 91(3): 591–594

McClung H J, Boyne L, Heitlinger L 1995 Constipation and dietary fibre intake in children. Pediatrics 96(5): 999–1001

Toiletting programmes

INTRODUCTION

Once the child's diet and laxative programme has been designed to the satisfaction of all concerned, other aspects of the treatment must be tackled. One such issue is the toiletting programme. This is obviously only appropriate to children who are old enough to have sufficient understanding to become toilet trained. Children under the age of 2 years who were not previously trained are not included in this part of the programme, although some aspects are useful for educating parents when the time for toilet training arrives. This aspect of treatment concentrates on teaching the child to use the toilet appropriately for bowel movements on a regular basis. Some children will be using the toilet successfully on occasion, but in between times will have soiling episodes; others will never have used the toilet successfully, and these patients are harder to cope with. Some will not have been taught to use the toilet; others do not recognise the signals from their body telling them it is time to go to the toilet. The first task of the health professional is to determine to which category the individual patient belongs; is it lack of training or ignorance of their own body causing this child's particular problem?

The assessment carried out at the first appointment will have given much of the information needed to decide what is required by this child. It may be that, as the child continues to attend the clinic and they and their parent become more relaxed in your presence, they will give further information on the problem. An open mind and receptive attitude towards disclosures of what actually happens at home is vital to encourage these trickles of facts about this child. It may take several appointments for the mother to tell you that this child has never sat on the toilet to defecate, as happened with one of the families seen at my own clinic. This young man was at nursery and was still wearing nappies. Some families appear to be so open they tell absolutely everything at the first meeting, but will open further as trust develops between themselves and the health professional managing their case. Part of the reason for this may concern their perception of what is acceptable to tell and what should not be disclosed to anyone. As they see the professional at a number of appointments and everything they say is treated with a non-judgmental response, it becomes safer to tell those 'secrets' not yet told to others. One mother who attended my clinic had told me things were very bad at home with her son's problem, but only when things had worsened following a hospital appointment with a consultant who had prescribed Picolax did she disclose that the child tended to soil all over the house. It appeared with closer questioning of the child that he had never responded to his body's signal of the urge to defecate, because he was not aware that he had to. He ignored any abdominal symptoms, and when the reflex stimulated by the Picolax became so strong that his bowels opened, it occurred wherever he happened to be. At times he would be in his bedroom, at others in the living-room. Mother stated that the house smelled appallingly and she was at her wit's end trying to cope with it. Had it not been for a sudden worsening of the situation, this mother might have waited even longer before she disclosed this particular situation, despite the fact that it was useful for the management of her son's condition.

These points remind us that assessment is an ongoing process and questions need to be asked at every appointment to clarify the situation for each individual child. Some information will be volunteered by the family; some will need further exploration to ascertain the true state of affairs. The atmosphere within the consultation has to be right to encourage the sharing of delicate information by the family. If a brusque, business-like attitude is presented to the family, it may prevent them from opening up to the health professional. If the professional tries to present an open, caring attitude to the family it may encourage them to share

---

Box 7.1   Points to remember

- Assessment is an ongoing process: check out at each visit how things are at home; other 'secrets' may come out as trust develops
- Ask questions of the child. Does he have abdominal pain, if so, what does he do when he gets it?
- Always present an open and non-judgmental attitude to whatever you are told. It may encourage vital information to be disclosed.

---

what may be vital information. Think which situation would be more likely to persuade you to disclose information about yourself!

ENVIRONMENT

When starting a toiletting programme, the room that the toilet is in should be considered. Is it welcoming? Is it very utilitarian? Help the parent to examine their toilet or bathroom with new eyes. Does the room encourage a child to stay in it for sufficient time to use the toilet effectively? Are there activities he can perform while sitting on the toilet? Is the room brightly decorated with pictures to look at? All of these can help with a toiletting programme.

One mother once told me her son was in and out of the bathroom in 30 seconds flat. In such a short timespan, there is no way he could effectively sit on the toilet to have his bowels open. Discussion on ways to encourage him to stay longer considered a cassette player, so he could listen to music or talking books; books to look at and read were decided upon. Mother also decided to put up posters for him to look at and to brighten the room.

Privacy is a great need for all of us when using the toilet. How many of us are happier to wait until getting home to our own toilet, rather than using a public convenience to empty our bowels? Children feel exactly the same. If the child is school-aged, it can be a particular problem. School toilets must be some of the worst places to use. They are often smelly and dirty, because children do not treat them with respect, and privacy can be a foreign word in them. As the doors and partitions do not reach the floor or ceiling there is always the possibility that another child will look under or over them, denying other children their much valued privacy. In many secondary schools, the situation can be even worse, as there may be no soap or towels available because other pupils have abused the facilities in the past. It is little wonder, then, that many children refuse to use the toilet at school, waiting until they reach home, even if it is detrimental to their health. Clayden (1996) agrees:

> Many children refuse to use these because the doors do not lock or the cubicles have wide gaps at the top or bottom of the walls and doors. Many children leave the lavatory in a disgusting state whereas others are afraid that they will leave behind a smell which will prove to others, and especially those who tease them, that they have recently defaecated. Children who are constipated and eventually open their bowels after several days of delay pass very offensive stools which amplify this problem.

The health professional may need to negotiate with the schools to ensure children have access to appropriate facilities if necessary. It would, however, be preferable for the child to attempt to time bowel evacuations for the morning before school, so that the home toilet can be used and to remove the dilemma of whether to use the school toilet at all.

While school and public toilets can be a specific problem for some children, the toilet at home can offer little privacy. If the toilet is in the bathroom, or if there are a number of children in the household, guaranteeing privacy can be almost impossible. In this situation, there has to be an agreement formed with the other members of the family concerning use of the toilet. A suitable time for the child with the soiling problem to have access to the toilet without interruption, to ensure effective participation in the management plan, should be agreed and adhered to.

Comfort is another aspect that affects the child's desire to remain in the toilet for sufficient time to perform adequately. The room being cold and unwelcoming will deter a child from staying there. If the seat is missing, or if the hole is too large to sit on without fear of losing balance and falling down the toilet, it can inhibit the wish to comply. Children have some endearingly funny ideas about toilets and what would happen to them if they were to fall down into them. If they have been frightened by someone flushing the toilet while they were sitting on it, this will be even worse and will have to be overcome first. So a comfortable seat that is the right size is vital. Inner seats for toilets are available from many stores selling baby equipment, at a reasonable price. These are ideal as they are designed to make the hole in the toilet seat

---

Box 7.2   Points to remember

- The toilet must give: comfort, privacy and be inviting to a child to encourage him to sit there
- School and public toilets are not nice places to visit
- Overcome fear by asking parents to use a doll to demonstrate sitting on the toilet

---

smaller so that younger children can sit on the seat comfortably. The use of a toilet step or bench to shorten the distance between seat and floor for the feet to rest on is also a good idea. Children will be able to sit quite still and the fear of falling down is removed as they can see the space is reduced. If the child is obviously scared that falling down the toilet is a real possibility, it may help to demonstrate with a doll that this is impossible. Using a doll or teddy to demonstrate sitting on the toilet can help in other ways too.

Where does 'poo' go?

Some children have very real concerns about their 'poo'. They worry about it going into the toilet and the fact that it disappears when the toilet is flushed. It is important to take the time to listen to these fears and alleviate them effectively. Brushing aside the fears is not sufficient; you must listen to them and explain in language they understand that 'poo' belongs in the toilet and when it is flushed down the pipe it goes to join other 'poos'. The first few times this is tried, it feels strange, but it soon becomes easier and the children come to trust an adult who talks to them in their own language. This is particularly true when that adult talks about things other adults usually ignore or prevaricate about. You can make up stories or use story books which are available in children's bookstores to help them to understand why 'poo' must go in the toilet. There are several good books around which are extremely useful for this and other aspects of the condition; it may be useful to build a small library of your own to show parents and children. The parents may then decide to buy their own copies of the books.

Taubman (1997) carried out a prospective study on children who refused to use the toilet to pass a stool, despite using it to pass urine. He looked at 482 children, between the ages of 18 and

---

Box 7.3 Points to remember

- Some children are afraid of toilets and where 'poo' goes
- Collect a library of books to illustrate toilets and 'poo' to show to children and parents
- Look at strategies for helping children overcome their fears

---

30 months, and found 22% of them had this problem. The factors found to be present were the presence of younger siblings and parental inability to set limits with those who had 'stool toiletting refusal'. He also found that these children had been potty trained later than the other children he looked at. Of the 106 children with stool toiletting refusal, 77 had no intervention and the problem spontaneously resolved within 6 months. For 28 children whose parents sought help from their paediatrician, he told parents to put the children back in nappies; 25 of them were using the potty within 3 months. Some children required a suppository, to stimulate evacuation, and a reward system. Although he was successful with the children he treated, there is no mention of why the children refused to sit on the potty for bowel movements. The same treatment would obviously not be appropriate for children older than those in his study. Putting children over the age of three and a half into nappies, particularly if they have not worn them for a long time, can be damaging to their self-esteem. It would almost certainly be impossible to overcome parental resistance to this method too.

How long?

One question often asked is for how long the child should sit on the potty or toilet. There are different schools of thought on this. Some think that the child should sit on the toilet for 1 minute for every year of their age, i.e. a five-year-old sits for 5 minutes and a ten-year-old for 10 minutes. Others believe very young children should sit for 5 minutes and school-aged for no longer than 10 minutes. As there is no real evidence to back either way of thinking, I suggest professionals choose whichever they feel more comfortable with, and stick with it. It may be that you might choose to alternate between the two different methods; the difficulty here is keeping in mind what you have told each child, unless you document clearly. I tend to favour the 5 and 10 minutes pattern,

---

Box 7.4   Points to remember

- There are two schools of thought on how long a child should sit on the toilet for. One says 1 minute for each year of the child's age, the other either 5 or 10 minutes
- Stick to one way or the other; try not to swap from one to the other
- Use a timing device to ensure accuracy

---

as it is straightforward and simple for parents to remember at a time when they are given so much information. The important thing is to ensure parents time the period the child spends on the toilet accurately. One mother told me her child altered the clock or timer she used for this. So another tip is to keep the timing device out of the child's reach but in easy view.

STIMULATING A GASTROCOLIC REFLEX

For the child to use the toilet successfully, he needs to experience the urge to defecate. While this may happen as an effect of the stimulant laxative, it should also be possible to stimulate it with certain foods and drinks. I often suggest that the school-aged child be given a cup of warm or hot tea to drink in the morning, and many parents have found this successful in stimulating the desire to open the bowels. Some people will respond better to ice-cold drinks or foods. Sometimes, a particular fruit or vegetable may be effective. For others, it may be a cereal-based food. For some it can take a lot of trial and error before the right food is found. Think about your own responses to certain foods; can you identify what causes you to have a noticeable gastrocolic reflex?

USING ABDOMINAL SYMPTOMS

Using the toilet for defecation successfully depends upon the child becoming aware of his own body. He needs to recognise what his body is telling him and what his response should be.

Box 7.5   Points to remember

- Some foods will stimulate a gastrocolic reflex
- Identify which work for each child
- Have a list of suggestions for the parents to try

This sounds simple, but it is surprising how many children do not know that our abdominal symptoms are telling us to go to the toilet. For these children, we need to spell out as simply as possible what they may experience and what their action must be. For some, this can be demonstrated with a stimulant laxative. The laxative is sometimes given in a sufficiently large dose to result in the abdominal cramps which precede the urge to defecate when the dose is being adjusted or a strong stimulant such as Picolax is prescribed. The parents and child must be told to expect these symptoms and that they serve to demonstrate the body's need to empty the bowels. They must also be given clear instructions on what to do when the symptoms occur. To reassure both parent and child, inform them that the dose of stimulant laxative will not always give these effects, as the dose will be lowered or the medication changed. Parents become anxious about this because they do not like to see their child in pain and the abdominal cramps can be quite severe, although they are usually short-lived and disappear once the bowels have been opened. Obviously, if the child has abdominal symptoms and responds appropriately to them, there is no need to explain this. However, they must be encouraged to respond to them every time.

Using either stimulant laxatives or a gastrocolic reflex effectively also helps to time bowel evacuations. Ideally, in the school-aged child, this should be in the morning before school so that the rectum is empty and is unlikely to need to be emptied again during the school day. To allow this, the timing of administration of the laxative or the food that precipitates a gastrocolic reflex needs careful adjustment. In Chapter 6 we saw that while senna takes between 18 to 24 hours to be effective, Picolax is much shorter acting. This may need changing as the child and parent grow accustomed to its action. So the time of administration may be earlier or later, dependent upon when the result happens and its convenience to the child and family.

Box 7.6   Points to remember

- Some children do not respond appropriately to abdominal symptoms
- They must be taught that this should precede a visit to the toilet
- Certain stimulant laxatives will cause abdominal pain

USEFUL AIDS

Before starting a toiletting programme, ask about the toilet facility at home and any special needs the child has. Although a seat insert has been discussed and should be used when appropriate, another helpful addition to bathroom furniture for young children is a toilet step or box. This gives children a 'counterbalance' of a stable surface for their feet to enable them to push effectively during defecation. The ability to push is much more difficult if one is also having to balance in mid-air.

Some conditions which result in poor spatial awareness, including cerebral palsy, can make using the toilet difficult because of the inability to sit upright in open space. If a child has this condition or another similar, and has toiletting difficulties, it is worthwhile looking at where the toilet is situated in the room. In a corner is the best location, but this is rarely the case. To counter the difficulty with spatial awareness, there are special frames available from specialist suppliers to fit around the toilet which give more stability and security to such children. Before investing in such frames test whether the child will benefit by using a large cardboard box cut to the appropriate size and shape to give some support to the child. Occupational therapists are experts at looking at the environment in which the child lives and suggesting appropriate adaptations; consult them if you have any doubts. You could also use the Disabled Living Foundation, who have branches around the country and have available many aids for those with special needs.

STAGED TOILETTING PROGRAMME

For all children with constipation and soiling, the programme will be in different stages, but some will need more stages than others, dependent upon their current situation. For the child who

---

Box 7.7   Points to remember

- Seat inserts are valuable to help remove the fear of falling into the toilet
- Toilet steps or a box provides a level surface for the feet to rest on and push against to aid in the squatting position
- Use other aids for children with special and specific needs
- Get advice from an occupational therapist
- Contact the Disabled Living Foundation as appropriate

can use the toilet on occasion, the programme will be reasonably simple, but for the child who will not or has not sat on the toilet it will require much more work on the parents' part. The programme is broken down into stages, always working towards certain goals. The goals must be achievable, but not currently being realised. For example, the child able to use the toilet but having accidents in his pants puts his pants in an agreed location. The child frightened of the toilet stands outside the room for an agreed length of time, etc.

During the description of a programme it will be presumed that the child does not currently use the toilet and wears a nappy and work from there; other children would enter the programme at the relevant stage.

As stated, the first stage is to remove the child's fear of the toilet by encouraging him to sit or stand outside the room with the door open for increasing lengths of time. During the next stage, the child has to enter the room and stay there for increasing lengths of time. These stages must be supported by a parent, possibly with activities to distract the child. The room, as discussed earlier, must be as inviting as possible to the child. Once the fear of the room is dispelled, the child can be encouraged to sit on the toilet, first of all without performing. Encouraging the child to flush the toilet and watch toilet tissue disappear helps at this stage to communicate that this is not an awful or frightening thing. The next stage will be to encourage the child to perform on the toilet; if a nappy is normally worn, the child sits on the toilet wearing a nappy.

At all stages the child needs lots of praise for achieving the goals set—see the section on rewards. When the child will happily perform on the toilet, albeit in a nappy, the next stage can be tried. This is achieved by cutting a hole in the nappy prior to putting it on, so that the stool goes directly into the toilet. The next stages involve gradually increasing the size of the hole, until there is little of the nappy left and the child feels confident about sitting on the toilet to pass a stool without asking for a nappy. Some children, particularly those with special needs, will require a longer effort at this stage than others to achieve their goal.

All children happy to use the toilet for both urine and stool must be helped to use it effectively. A routine must be established using, as discussed, the laxatives, gastrocolic reflex and abdominal symptoms. It may be that in the beginning of the plan, when the child is first learning to respond to bodily signals, time is allowed for sitting on the toilet for an agreed period after each meal. As the desired result is achieved with laxatives and gastro-colic reflex, the child needs to try less frequently. Loening-Baucke (1997) states: 'Toilet-sitting frequency was reduced to once a day once the child felt the urge to defecate and initiated toilet use on his or her own.' For the child's sake, it is often best if the stool is passed in the morning to help prevent any leakage of faecal matter later in the day while out of the house. Loening-Baucke (1997) concurs: '...in the morning was that the bowel clean-out was accomplished before leaving for school and soiling was rare.' It may be that another stool will be passed in the evening until the laxative regime is tuned to the child's needs.

The child must have sufficient time to sit on the toilet and perform. This may mean that family routines have to alter to accommodate the child's needs. If everyone in the family gets up at the last minute before leaving for the day for school or work, the toilet or bathroom may not be free for a long enough time period for the child who soils. It may require an adult to rise earlier to wake the child and allow him to use the toilet first in the morning. It may require changes to other family members' routines to allow the time needed. These points should be discussed at length and options should be explored while the child and parent are with the health professional. If necessary, the child and parent may need to rehearse their responses to objections from other family members. To prepare their answer prior to the event helps them to deal effectively with arguments when and if they arise. When properly convinced of the benefits, other members of the family can be an asset in supporting the management plan. If unprepared, they may become resentful and hinder the execution of the plan.

It is important that a record of the child's progress is kept; the soiling baseline chart shown in Chapter 3 will effectively document the child's attempts to pass a stool in the toilet, any accidents and the child's concordance with the laxative regime. These charts will provide a graphic illustration of the child's progress so that both parent and child can look back and see just what has been achieved. This is important because, as the management of cases of chronic constipation takes a very long time, families can forget exactly what the patient was doing a month or more ago. They will become disheartened at times and the ability to demonstrate how far the child has progressed is vital to encourage continuation.

This preliminary discussion has covered issues that may be raised at home, how long the child will attempt to sit on the toilet and the regime of laxatives and their effect on toiletting. The need for changes to family routine has been explored, and how these will be accomplished. We have discussed how the child can be encouraged to use any relevant symptoms to time going to the toilet.

A toiletting programme is decided upon. At the start of treatment the child will sit on the toilet for 5–10 minutes depending upon age, and method preferred, after each meal. As the management plan becomes more settled and the laxatives stimulate a daily bowel evacuation, the child visits the toilet accordingly. As it is preferable to have a morning evacuation, the time of administration of the stimulant laxative will be adjusted until the result is at a time convenient for the child and family. A morning bowel evacuation is in common with a large number of the general population, who empty their bowels shortly after eating breakfast. Egg-timers and kitchen timers may help the parents to be certain the child is sitting on the toilet for a sufficient period. When building up to the agreed time, or with very young children, it may help to use a sand-filled egg-timer, as it will keep their attention and help to ease boredom.

REWARDS

Rewards are an integral part of the management plan in any situation which aims to change behaviour. For these children, we

---

Box 7.8 Points to remember

- Break the task down into small steps and set these as goals
- Although the ultimate goal is having full bowel control, this is not achievable straight away
- Set goals that are achievable
- The family may need to change their routines; rehearse responses to possible objections at the clinic
- Use symptoms, whether generated by laxatives or by gastrocolic reflex to time toilet visits
- Use a timer of some sort to time toilet use accurately
- Use charts to record the child's progress

need to change their toiletting behaviour and encourage appropriate use of the toilet for defecation. For any behaviour modification programme, there are some golden rules to follow if an
increased chance of success is sought. Any psychology text book
will give these golden rules when discussing behaviour modification.

Rule one

The first rule is that any goals that the child has to work towards
have to be achievable. The ultimate goal is to have the child with
complete bowel control and no more soiling. To put this as the
first step is dooming everyone to failure; it is simply not achievable at the beginning. By breaking this down into small steps, we
can help the child to progress towards the ultimate goal. Perhaps
the first goal will be that the child places soiled clothing in an
agreed place, or if this is already being done, that the child sits on
the toilet for an agreed time period after each meal. When this is
achieved routinely, another goal is set, with the agreement of both
child and parent. There are many small goals that can be used:
taking the medication at set times, eating fibre-rich foods, drinking the required number of drinks daily or, later in the programme, passing a stool in the toilet. These goals must be agreed
between health professional, child and parent at clinic appointments. At each subsequent visit, it is important that the child's
progress is examined and praise lavished on both child and parent. The child cannot achieve the goals without support from the
parent and therefore the parent needs a reward in the form of
praise from the health professional. Goal achievement can be
recorded on charts; personally I prefer not to use those with days
on as they can become a record of failure, (see Fig. 7.1). 'Road'
charts which have spaces to be coloured and a 'bridge' after 7 or
so spaces, at which time the child receives a reward previously
agreed, are much better and more adaptable, as the desired
behaviour may be achieved more than once a day.

Rule two

The reward should be negotiated between the child and parent,
but it has to be something the child will value. While a child aged
3 to 5 or 6 years may value a star on a chart, it is unlikely an older

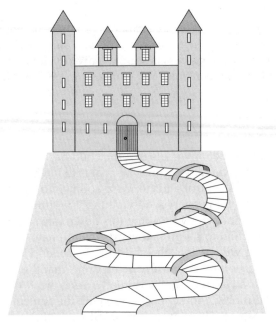

Figure 7.1 Reward chart: 'Road chart'.

child would. Rewards do not have to be of monetary value, although a small toy or book may be a nice treat now and then. Spending an extra half-hour with one or other parent, or another adult, choosing the evening meal for the family, visiting a local park to play on the swings are all effective rewards. Do try, however, not to help decide upon something that is not advisable. Agreeing on a visit to the local burger bar as a reward is not a good idea as it reinforces poor dietary habits early in the programme. If possible, give rewards at the clinic, particularly towards the end of treatment. Gathering a few small gifts that children can choose from at their final visit has great benefits.

Rule three

Any reward must be given immediately. In effect, that means the same day, not at the end of the week or when children are completely in control of their bowels. Many parents dangle large expensive treats for children to aim for and while, for some, this is effective, most children lose interest when their progress seems so slow and their chances of achieving the reward slip further away. So the value of small treats now becomes apparent; the child must get something for achieving the desired behaviour.

Rule four

The reward must be given *only* for the desired behaviour. The parent and child must understand that the reward is for achieving the goal set at the clinic. If the goal is achieved ten times before the next appointment, a reward should be given ten times. The parent must not succumb to any pressure put on them by the child or other members of the family to give the reward for other actions. If a reward is earned then another form of prize must be given for it.

Rule five

Once given, the reward should never be taken away again. If the desired behaviour has been achieved and rewarded, it is important there are not changes to this. If the reward is taken away, it may harm the behaviour modification programme immensely. If other behaviour requires sanctions to be imposed, they must not be related to the programme being undertaken. If the child achieves certain behaviour and then next time cannot, the failure must be ignored. There must be no punishments for failure to achieve a goal, even if it has previously been reached. It is well known that all individuals learn more from praise than from punishment, and the reinforcement given by rewarding the desired behaviour is vital. Removal of the same reward is a punishment that should not be considered. It gives the message that the previous achievement is not valued any longer.

With careful negotiation between all the players in this management plan, a reward system can be very effective, as long as the golden rules are adhered to. As the programme continues, the goals will be changed. While for a short time after the ultimate goal has been achieved, the rewards continue to be given, they will tail off. One big problem is convincing parents who do not believe the child should be rewarded for something they feel is 'normal' behaviour anyway. It will take a very persuasive argument on the health professional's part to explain why and how

---

Box 7.9 Points to remember

Rewards can be very effective as long as the golden rules are followed:

1. The goals must be achievable.
2. The reward must be valued by the child and negotiated between parent and child.
3. The reward must be given immediately.
4. The reward must only be given for the desired behaviour.
5. The reward should never be taken back once given.

---

this will work. A starting point has to be to convince them that their child does not soil clothing deliberately; with a full explanation of the condition, this should be possible.

REFERENCES

Clayden G 1996 A guide for good practice: childhood constipation. Ambulatory Child Health 1(5): 250–255

Loening-Baucke V 1997 Urinary incontinence and urinary tract infection and their resolution with treatment of chronic constipation of childhood. Pediatrics 100(2): 228–232

Taubman B 1997 Toilet training and toiletting refusal for stool only: a prospective study. Pediatrics 99(1): 54–58

8

Management: Stage 3

WITHDRAWAL OF TREATMENT

Introduction

The child and his family should, following completion of the management plan, now be at the stage where the withdrawal of active treatment can be considered. Felt et al (1999) tell us that children with 'idiopathic constipation and soiling usually require maintenance therapy for 6 to 24 months.' The length of time depends to some extent upon how long they have had the condition. A child who has been referred appropriately after suffering for only a few months is likely to need the maintenance therapy for a considerably shorter timespan than the child who has suffered since infancy and is referred at 7 years of age. There must be some set criteria for starting the withdrawal of treatment. Felt et al (1999) suggest: 'Recovery is defined as 3 or more stool productions per week with no soiling. Stool frequency of less than 3 per week with or without soiling indicates the need to continue with the maintenance programme.' These are very definite success or failure of treatment categories, and are easily followed in practice if records of toilet use and administration of laxatives are completed and returned to the health professional by the family on the soiling baseline chart. However, others would suggest that daily doses of stimulant laxatives should result in a daily stool production and this should be used as a criterion for considering withdrawal of treatment. As the aim of management is to reduce the volume of faeces required to stimulate the urge to defecate, a daily bowel evacuation is probably a good indication that this has been achieved.

Local agreement on the definition of success is vital before starting to treat children. As Felt et al are practitioners in the USA and their management differs a little from that used in the UK, I tend to go with the idea of daily evacuation as a measure of success. If a child is not having a daily bowel movement, the laxative regime probably needs some adjustment to achieve this. Loening-Baucke (1994 in Kamm) suggests: 'Laxatives need to be continued for several months and sometimes years at the right dose to induce daily soft stools.' However, she later states:

Clinical follow-up studies, usually 12 months after the start of treatment, show that 50% of children with chronic constipation will be off all laxative and have no recurrence of their symptoms. Another 20% may be weaned off within two years. The remainder will require laxatives for daily bowel movements for many years and occasionally into adulthood.

When the right time arrives for an individual child, it is vital that both child and parent are prepared. They should be warned that there may be times of relapse and that it may take anything from 6 to 12 months to completely wean the child off the laxatives. A full explanation of the process will inform them why it will take so long and why it is important that this is carried out slowly. The laxatives will be reduced in small steps, one at a time. This is important for the health professional because if both are reduced simultaneously and a problem arises, there is no way of knowing which laxative reduction has caused it. It is vital to highlight the need to continue other aspects of the treatment both during this process and afterwards. The changes made to dietary and fluid intake should ensure a regular soft stool, even in the absence of laxatives.

When?

As suggested already, when the child has been passing a regular daily soft stool for an agreed period of time is the right time to

---

Box 8.1 Points to remember

- There must be a 'weaning off' process which may be started between 6 to 12 months after maintenance therapy starts
- Recovery is defined as having 3 or more stool productions per week according to Felt et al. However, a daily passage of stool is preferable

stop treatment, as far as the constipation is concerned. When planning to see this group of children, it is important that policies are set first so that there is standardisation of when the weaning off will be attempted. There may be a blanket decision that every child will start weaning off laxatives after 6 months of daily soft stool production. There may be a case for a sliding scale of time periods. If a child has suffered for 1 year, he will start weaning after 6 months; if he has had it for 2 years it will be 9 months; after 3 years it will start after 12 months, etc. The policy may be written so that each case is assessed on the merit of the clinical symptoms and progress. Without some written policy, however, each child has an almost pot-luck chance on the introduction of specific stages of management. This is obviously far from ideal for the child or the parent.

The family life also needs to be taken into account. If there is any change or stressful time expected, it is best to avoid trying to start weaning off laxatives. Similarly, if the health professional is not going to be available for a week or two because of leave, it is much better to delay starting the process. Loening-Baucke (1997) states: 'after regular bowel habits were established for several months, the laxative dose was gradually decreased to a dose that maintained one bowel movement daily and prevented soiling.'

Why?

The reason that weaning is considered is to ensure the child does not rely on laxatives for longer than is necessary. It is never advisable to maintain long-term use of any medication if it can be avoided, and in most cases of chronic constipation in children it can be avoided. The aim of the management is to restore normal physiological function of the bowel and, by using laxatives, to stimulate the passing of a soft daily stool. If physiologically normal function has been restored, the laxatives should be superfluous. The vast majority of children never use laxatives at all and,

---

Box 8.2   Points to remember

- When child is passing at least one daily soft stool
- Avoid any emotional upheaval in the family, if possible
- Time the start of the process for when the health professional will be available for support

---

Box 8.3 Points to remember

- Once normal physiological function has been restored, the laxatives should be discontinued
- If they are not discontinued, normal physiological function cannot be proved
- Longer term use of any medication is not recommended if it is no longer necessary

---

in order that the children with constipation and soiling rejoin that majority, it is important that they too do not rely on laxatives for any longer than is necessary. Look in almost any drug book at entries for laxatives, and they will state that laxatives are not recommended for long-term use. While they have been used long-term for this group of children, they have now performed the task for which they were introduced. There now needs to be a testing time to ascertain whether this change will be maintained without the help of laxatives.

How?

As stated, this must be carried out slowly to maintain a daily bowel evacuation while reducing the dose of laxative. The need to reduce one laxative at a time has been discussed. It is vital that parent and child have access to the health professional during this time, so a contact number should be given. If running a clinic forms only a part of your role, a convenient number where staff will take a message that you check in with daily should be set up. During the weaning, parents and child will feel particularly vulnerable and will need support from 'their' trusted health professional. Even if another colleague has similar expertise to the health professional they have seen, they will not have the same trust in their advice. 'Their' health professional knows them fully and understands their problem and another member of staff is not good enough for them at this trying time.

While a contact number is important, regular appointments must also be made at this time. It may be necessary to give weekly appointments after the first reduction in medication, but as time goes on they can be timed to coincide with the next reduction. This will vary from one health professional to another. Loening-Baucke (1997) reports: 'After 3 months, a further reduction until discontinuation of laxatives was attempted. Treatment resumed if constipation recurred.' Others might suggest a reduction in dose every 2 to 3 weeks. There must be local agreement on the time between each reduction when the clinic is first arranged. This, again, is something that should be included in local policy before a clinic is set up. The frequency of the clinic may influence choice of time between reductions. If the clinic is a weekly event, this is the best option, as timespans can be decided upon by clinical evidence. Some will be every fortnight, others monthly, and this will limit the time between reductions to 2, 4 or 6 weeks or at monthly intervals.

Each reduction is very small, at only 0.5 ml at each step. As mentioned, one laxative is reduced at a time, however before it is completely stopped the dose may remain static and the other laxative may be reduced. This may be repeated on several occasions until the first laxative is reduced further, until it is stopped, and then the same repeated with the other laxative. The laxative chosen to start with is often down to the personal choice of the health professional, but symptoms may indicate which to start with. If there is abdominal pain and the child is passing more than one stool each day, the stimulant would be the one to begin reducing. If the child is passing a very soft stool daily, the stool softener is chosen first. If at any time in the weaning off period the symptoms recur, the dose is increased back to the previous successful reduced dose. At this point, it may be that the other laxative is slowly reduced while continuing this same dose. The first laxative may then be reduced again to see if problems recur.

Box 8.4   Points to remember

- Reduction must be done slowly in small steps, 0.5 ml at each reduction
- One laxative at a time only; otherwise if there are problems it is difficult to know which one has caused them
- The first may be reduced only halfway, before halting and starting to reduce the other
- Reductions are timed every 3 weeks to 3 months, dependent on local policy
- Diet and fluid intake must be maintained
- Support must be available from the health professional managing the case

AVOIDING PITFALLS

Education

For some children, there will undoubtedly be problems when the dose of their laxatives is reduced. Sometimes it is because psychologically they feel that, unless they take the medication, they will return to their old problem. As they have now found a new lease of life without it, they do not want the constipation and soiling to return. It may be the parent who has a problem accepting that the child will be able to manage bowel control without the help of their laxatives. If they are remembering the situation prior to treatment, they may worry that it will recur. Remember, these medications have been part of their daily routine for a long time now. They may be used as a crutch by both the child and the parent. It will take skilful explanation on the part of the health professional to ensure this weaning off is completed with as few problems as possible. Some thought put into the planning of the weaning process can pay dividends for both the child and the parent, and the health professional. Preparing the child mentally, with education and by ensuring the correct time is identified for the process to start are both vital first steps in helping to guarantee a good chance of success.

Throughout the previous sections in this text, it has been emphasised how important the education of both the child and the parents on the condition and management is, and the role this will play in the success of the management plan. When the management reaches the weaning stage, it is vital to ensure that the child and parent will comply with the planned reduction and will continue to trust the health professional. This will also help them to avoid some of the potential problems that may occur at this time. If they are aware of what may happen and how to deal with potential problems, they will confront the situation much more confidently. If they are not given advance notice of what may happen, they may start to think they have failed and that no-one else has had the same problems. This can be catastrophic for their self-esteem, and when this has probably only recently recovered from previous knocks caused by the constipation and soiling, this is to be avoided if at all possible. It can also cause problems for the professional trying to manage the condition, as the weaning off will be seen as an inappropriate move on the professional's part.

So, as someone once said, education, education, education is the key to success. The more the child and parent can be taught about the problem, the better. This is not a case of a little knowledge being a dangerous thing, nor of ignorance being bliss. This is a case of forewarned is forearmed! While telling the child and parent what they are to do and why it is important, it is much better practice to have the details written down so they can take it away with them to consult as necessary. The use of printed pro-forma for this type of information, which the health professional can complete with doses, etc. is a valuable tool to save time in the consultation.

Timing

Correct timing of the process is another key to helping ensure success. This has been discussed earlier but its importance cannot be over-emphasised. There has to be a good chance of success when the weaning off begins, or the child's self-esteem will take another beating. So choose a time when it is fairly certain that the child's rectum has returned to a physiologically normal size. This is obviously not something that can be ascertained by looking at the patient; the size and frequency of the stools are the only clue that will be apparent. If the problem has been present in a child for a number of years, it is going to take a very long time before the rectum has had the chance to recover its normal size. Two years or more on maintenance and weaning is not unusual in this type of case. A younger child who has had the problem for less than a year will probably still need maintenance for a number of months before considering weaning. If the child is ready physically, and has had lots of education about the weaning process and why it must be done, plan when it will start.

Look at what is happening in the child's life and in the family. If there is any upheaval at present or any anticipated in the near future, such as a house move, a new baby due or a marital split, etc., delay starting until these have passed and life has settled again. A good time may be considered to be in the school holidays with a school-aged child. This is not so good, however, if the family is going away, maybe even abroad, where accessing help may be difficult, if not impossible.

Support at this time, as already mentioned, is vital, so access to the health professional managing the case must be available. If the health professional has other duties there must be a messaging system set up. If this is not feasible, the health professional must contact the family by telephone if possible or, if not, by making a

---

Box 8.5 Points to remember

- Pitfalls in the weaning process can be avoided if careful planning is undertaken
- Get the timing for starting right
- Ensure plenty of support is available
- Give a thorough explanation of the process and its importance
- Local policy should be developed on aspects of the management of weaning off laxatives
- Good quality written information to back up the verbal instructions is valuable
- Warn both the child and parent of potential problems—forewarned is forearmed

---

home visit. Examine all avenues to ensure both child and parents have access to sufficient expert advice during a time when they will feel very uncertain about the management plan. It may be that the family will sail through the weaning process without a single problem but this is very unusual; many families will have a problem of some sort. The problems will vary from minor ones, including forgetting the instructions or losing written information, to major problems like a total failure to pass a stool after the first dosage reduction. Whatever the problem, the family will feel it is a major catastrophe and will want to talk to their health professional to obtain advice. Unless health professionals work in total isolation, a system for taking and passing on messages is usually fairly simple to arrange.

This brings to mind another point which was briefly covered earlier. If the health professional who has managed the case is not going to be available to give the required support, it is worth waiting until they are.

RECOGNISING PROBLEMS

While a good number of the children who attend clinics for help with this condition will have few problems with the weaning off process, some will have more serious problems. As a health professional managing their case, it is important that you can recognise when things are going wrong and know what to do about it.

For most children, the first sign that there is a problem will be when they fail to produce a daily stool. While not having the bowels open every day is perfectly acceptable among the general population, it has to be noted early in the children being discussed. Again, recording the medications the child takes and the stool frequency is a vital tool in assessing their progress while weaning. Missing one day every now and then is not a problem, but if the child passes fewer than three stools in any one week, the weaning process must be halted and returned to the previous step.

If the child or parents report an increase in flatulence, a careful check on progress is a good idea. Increased flatulence may indicate there is a slowing down in colonic motility. Digested food is staying longer in the colon, with the result that the gut flora have longer to work on the contents and to produce more gas. If the colon slows down and these symptoms are noted, it may be that in the near future there may be a harder stool because more water is absorbed which could potentially start the whole cycle again. As the stool is staying in the colon longer and drying out further, it will also be slightly smaller and the volume required to stimulate the defecation reflex would not be reached in the rectum. A failure to stimulate this reflex results in the need for a larger faecal mass to arouse it.

It is important, therefore, that both child and parents are made aware of the need for caution if they spot any potential problems such as increased flatulence or abdominal pain. Abdominal pain may result from the colon working harder to expel the faecal matter. Children will often describe the pain as coming and going or not being there all the time. Adults would describe it as cramping or intermittent, and this is because the colonic activity is increased to move the contents along to the rectum and start the defecation reflex. Along with the abdominal pain, there may be a degree of abdominal distension. This is an obvious sign that there are problems arising from the reduced dose of laxative. The constipation is obviously returning with this new lower dose and the health professional must therefore take some action to prevent real problems.

Once the step backwards on the weaning off process has been taken, it is sensible to allow the child a little time to settle at this new lower than previous maintenance dose. Some practitioners suggest a 6-month break before trying to wean off again, and using the same process, others would suggest a shorter time. It may be that at this time this laxative is left at the lower dose and the other laxative is reduced slowly. If the problems arise again, the most judicious thing to do is to keep both at the minimum dose that can safely be given while maintaining a daily bowel evacuation. Other

---

Box 8.6 Points to remember

- Early recognition of problems is vital
- Failure to produce a daily stool on two consecutive days must be investigated by talking to the child or parent
- Reported increase in flatulence is not a good sign. Colonic motility may be reduced
- Abdominal symptoms such as griping pains or distension should not be ignored
- Any symptoms that indicate problems should result in the return to the previous dose upon which there were no symptoms
- The other laxative may be reduced at this time, but slowly
- It may be necessary to halt all reductions for a time and try again at a later date

---

aspects of the management plan must be continued, i.e. the diet and fluid intake and any toiletting routine that was set up.

Both the child and the parent will require much reassurance if problems occur and the weaning off process is halted for a time. They need to be convinced that this is a minor hiccup and that the weaning off will restart once his bowel becomes accustomed to the lower dose. Obviously, when it is decided the time is right to start the weaning off process again, the same preparation must be made. It may prove a little more difficult to persuade the child and the parent that this will work this time and that trying to reduce is the correct thing to do. The effort must be made, however, because the child must be allowed to try without laxatives if at all possible. If at any time the health professional managing the case has concerns about the progress of an individual child, they should consult a more experienced colleague, or a paediatrician, or the child's general practitioner for support in the case.

REFERENCES

Felt B, Wise C G, Olson A, Kochlar P, Marcus S, Coran A 1999 Guideline for the management of pediatric idiopathic constipation and soiling. Archives of Pediatric Adolescent Medicine 153(Apr): 380–385

Kamm M A, Lennard-Jones J E 1994 Constipation. Wrightson Biomedical Publishing, Petersfield

Loening-Baucke V 1997 Urinary incontinence and urinary tract infection and their resolution with treatment of chronic constipation of childhood. Pediatrics 100(2): 228–232

9

Good practice

The previous chapters in this text have alluded to some areas of good practice; this chapter aims to bring them all together. There are different aspects to what can be considered good practice— some are clinical, some professional and others are legal requirements. Each health professional has a code of professional conduct to adhere to. This text will not be exploring these as such, but will try to focus on the broader issues applicable to all those who seek to help and support children with chronic constipation and soiling. For obvious reasons, any quotes supporting the argument will be from the UKCC Code of Conduct or other publications by the professional body.

All health professionals should be following best evidence in clinical practice; however, there is very little available concerning constipation and soiling in children. A literature search will provide a number of articles and small research projects on specific areas of the subject but none that cover the management from day one to the end. There are a number of reasons for this and perhaps the most important one is that many of the drugs used are not big money-makers for the manufacturers. The licence for the laxatives in common use are no longer in the sole ownership of one company and, because the profit from them is small, the funds for research are non-existent.

Every living organism feeds and they all excrete in one way or another. This does not, however, make it an attractive area on which to concentrate one's expertise. As it is not a glamorous area, it attracts little funding from research organisations which are more likely to donate to areas of medicine that deal with life-threatening conditions. While this results in there being little practical evidence for a practitioner to use, it is no excuse to give a poor service to one's clients. There are practitioners who have devoted a great deal of their professional lives to looking after these children and now have policies that are clinically effective in the management of chronic constipation and soiling which should be used to build local policies.

I have heard a speaker (a national expert in the field) tell an audience that constipation seems to have become more prevalent since the advent of sell-by dates. Why? Before sell-by dates people would, on occasion, eat food that was past its best and as a result would have a touch of diarrhoea which would clear the bowel and remove any faecal mass. Since, as a society, we have become more careful about food because of food production scares, other problems have arisen. Solving one problem often leads to others. In managing these children, all we can do is the best possible with the current evidence. Some things will help in the delivery of the best care while others will hinder. What follows is an entirely personal view of what constitutes good practice.

STAFF

My own personal view is that no-one should be coerced into managing the children with whom this book is concerned. They deserve someone who is interested in them and their condition. Some authorities feel that everyone should manage this group of children whether they are interested or not. These children need someone who is enthusiastic about their management and is

---

Box 9.1 Points to remember

- There are different aspects to good practice: clinical, professional and legal
- Codes of professional conduct should be followed by individual practitioners
- There is little all-encompassing research to follow for best evidence
- Experts in the field have developed policies for managing children with constipation and soiling

knowledgeable about the condition and its management. To gain knowledge, health professionals have to be prepared to read and research the areas that are of specific interest to them. Alternatively, they can attend conferences and study days on the condition, if they are being held. All practitioners have a duty to keep up-to-date as part of lifelong learning. The UKCC (2001) tells us: 'Lifelong learning is more than simply keeping up to date. It requires an enquiring approach to the practice of nursing, midwifery and health visiting, as well as to issues which impact on that practice.' As a nurse, I follow the UKCC Code of Conduct (1992) which exhorts nurses to 'maintain and improve your professional knowledge and competence' and to 'acknowledge any limitations in your knowledge and competence and decline any duties or responsibilities unless able to perform them in a safe and skilled manner.' Many other codes of conduct have similar phrases that suggest that unless the professional is trained in a specific area, the task should not be undertaken and that any knowledge the practitioner has should be as up-to-date as possible.

Along with staff being knowledgeable and enthusiastic, they need to be sympathetic to the child and the parents' plight. They must be able to support these families adequately by listening to the problems and giving advice that will help. Some of the things that both the child and parent will tell the health professional can be quite shocking. The health professional must present an open manner and a non-judgmental attitude to all they are told. It may be that the parental attitude to the problem has in the past been questionable, but if they now present a positive attitude to supporting their child through their condition they need the praise and support of those working with them. This statement does not mean that past child abuse should be ignored. All health professionals have a duty to protect children, and should follow local policies and procedures for child protection.

The description of the staff who should be managing these cases will cause some local problems. If, for example, only one member of a team of nurses or health visitors is interested in managing the children with constipation and soiling, they may receive referrals from their colleagues. The colleagues should therefore be willing to 'pay back' the time taken with these children by offering support in other areas of the caseload. Obviously, this will depend upon local arrangements and professional courtesy.

Box 9.2 Points to remember

- All staff who manage these children should be enthusiastic and motivated
- All health professionals have a duty to keep up-to-date about their current areas of practice
- Staff must be sympathetic and present a non-judgmental attitude
- Local policies on child protection must be adhered to
- Local arrangements are necessary to support the staff managing children with constipation and soiling

---

HISTORY AND ASSESSMENT

Without a thorough history being taken and a full assessment being completed, any treatment plan designed around an individual child is less likely to succeed. The history-taking and assessment procedures covered in Chapter 3 provide all staff with the basic information required to assess, plan, implement and evaluate any care to be delivered to a child with constipation and soiling. These four steps should form the basis of any care package designed for any individual and in any situation. If only half the information is available to the health professional, it makes planning a programme of care like trying to bake a cake with only half the ingredients. The result is somewhat disappointing and unexpected.

BASELINE CHARTS

Although they form an integral part of an assessment, the use of baseline charts is another indication for me that good practice is being followed. The reasons for using baseline charts have been mentioned previously. They form a written record of the starting point for the child. They are useful for comparison when judging progress. Perhaps most importantly they can be

---

Box 9.3 Points to remember

- A thorough history and complete assessment are vital to any care given to these children
- Using a well-designed assessment form can aid the process
- There are four steps in care giving: assessing, planning, implementing and evaluating

---

Box 9.4   Points to remember

- Baseline charts form an integral part of the assessment
- They can provide a point for comparison
- They can demonstrate progress to child and parent

---

used to demonstrate to both the child and the parent how far they have progressed, particularly when they become disheartened.

REGULAR FOLLOW-UP

Although it can be argued that once every 6 months constitutes regular follow-up, for these children it is not often enough. They need almost weekly appointments at the beginning of treatment and at other times throughout the management of their condition. It may be that at other times they will be seen less frequently. After any change made to their management plan they should be offered another appointment within 2 weeks. Muir & Burnett (1999) agree:

In order to achieve successful management of childhood constipation, families require a consistent and supportive approach. Follow-up needs to be regular, with the provision of sufficient time to identify and explore their needs holistically.

If appointments are a problem, support over the telephone must be made available for the clients at any clinic. For many paediatricians and general practitioners this need for regular, fairly lengthy appointments can be problematic, and for this reason other health professionals are often a better alternative to manage the case.

Box 9.5   Points to remember

- Appointments may be required at weekly intervals at the start of management and at times of changes to management
- As child and parent become more confident in the management, the intervals between appointments can be lengthened
- If appointments are not available, contact with the family must be achieved through another medium

---

WHEN TO GET HELP

The practitioner who is aware that the problems of an individual child are beyond their own expertise, and takes steps to refer on to someone who is able to manage the case effectively is exhibiting good practice. Often the problem is that there is no-one else who is better able to manage the case locally. Use what resources are available. If there is a local continence advisor, whether they treat children or not, they have expertise in the area and can at the very least give some guidance on where to go for help. It may be that the health professional has to invest time into improving their own knowledge about a particular aspect of management in order to give the correct advice and support to a child. Perhaps finding out about others locally who have expertise in the condition prior to starting to see these children is a good idea.

CONSENT

While consent may be implied because the child and parent have attended the appointment sent to them, legally consent must be sought for any treatment. Involving children in discussions about their management can be one step towards ensuring that any consent gained is informed. For the vast majority of the treatment, this implied and verbal consent that children give when they agree to try certain parts of their management plan is sufficient. However some of the investigations and some treatments during the first stage of the management—the bowel evacuation—will require informed written consent. The Department of Health (2001) has recently issued guidelines on consent to treatment and examination which state:

For consent to be valid, it must be given voluntarily by an appropriately informed person (the patient or where relevant someone with parental responsibility for a patient under the age of 18) who has the capacity to

---

Box 9.6 Points to remember

- Investigate local 'experts' before seeing children
- Often there is no other professional seeing these children
- Use the resources that are available, e.g. continence advisors have knowledge about constipation and may have access to others who treat children

---

Box 9.7 Points to remember

- Consent is required for any invasive treatment or investigations
- To be legal, it must be given voluntarily and be based upon the information given
- Parental consent is required for children, although the child may then refuse that consent if they are *Gillick competent*
- Although written consent is not taken at each visit, by negotiating any changes to treatment, implied consent is obtained

---

consent to the intervention in question. Acquiescence where the person does not know what the intervention entails is not "consent".

While many of the children seen at clinics for constipation and soiling will need consent from the parent with parental responsibility it must be remembered that under the *Gillick* ruling, more mature children may be assessed to be competent to give and withhold consent to treatment.

Good practice would always seek consent by negotiating steps of the management plan with both child and parent, whether any intervention is required by the health professional or not. Having alternatives available if the first treatment option is not suitable for the individual child and family is an integral part of the negotiating process.

POLICIES, PROTOCOLS AND PATIENT GROUP DIRECTIVES

When a decision is taken to start seeing children with chronic constipation and soiling, whether as part of the individual health professional's caseload or by running a clinic, it is vital that policies and procedures are written first. The number of policies and procedures will vary from one setting to another, and depending whether the clinic is nurse-led or doctor-led. Muir & Burnett (1999) tell us:

A priority in setting up the nurse led clinic was the establishment of a consistent protocol for the management of intractable childhood constipation. This protocol was based on research evidence, policy directives and clinical experience.

It is at this time that all forms and other stationery can be designed, if they are not already available. This process can be time-consuming but the preparation will pay dividends later if the clinic is to run smoothly and no obstacles to managing a case are to be encountered. Think through the scope of practice within the management of these cases that will be carried out by the health professional: this will give the areas requiring a policy. It may be that the clinic is designed so that all children see a paediatrician first for investigations and are then sent to the nurse-led clinic for their management. Policies in this instance would be couched in terms that require the child to be assessed by a doctor first. It may be that the management is carried out in the community with support from a community paediatrician or the children's general practitioners. In this case, it may be that there is a protocol for the nurse to refer for certain investigations.

By far the most common policy and protocol will be around the use of laxatives: what will be used as a first choice, when any changes can be made to dose or type and what will be second option, etc. This is, in effect, a Patient Group Directive which the review group led by Dr June Crown (Department of Health 1998) defined thus:

A Group Protocol is a specific written instruction for the supply or administration of named medicines in an identified clinical situation. It is drawn up locally by doctors, pharmacists and other appropriate professionals and approved by the employer, advised by the relevant professional committees. It applies to groups of patients or other service users who may not be individually identified before presentation for treatment.

Since this time, the name for group protocols has been changed legally to Patient Group Directives. Of course, since this was formulated some groups of nurses can now prescribe drugs, and laxatives would be included in the *Nurse Prescribers' Formulary* which is incorporated into the BNF. Very recently, there were also changes to allow more nurses to train to be nurse prescribers and to use a wider *Formulary*. While this will help when managing those children with constipation and soiling, it is still important to have guidelines for clinics about dosage required and about when to refer back to a doctor for more complicated cases. Many laxatives are on the General Sale List which the UKCC (2000) describes as: 'These need neither a prescription nor the supervision of a pharmacist and can be obtained from retail outlets.' They further state, concerning this group of medicines:

Generally, no medication should be administered without a prescription. However, local policies or patient group directions should be developed to

---

Box 9.8 Points to remember

- Policies, protocols and procedures should be written before starting to see children with constipation and soiling
- Patient group directives require the signature of a doctor and pharmacist to ratify them; there are suggested formats for these documents
- The number of policies should be decided locally after examining what the particular professional will manage and what will be managed by others
- Preparing these in advance will help to ensure a smoother clinic for the professional and the clients

---

allow limited administration of medicines in this group to meet the needs of patients.

Muir & Burnett (1999) write on this:

A standardised approach to the administration of agreed medication under group protocol arrangements. A multidisciplinary group was formed in order to identify named medicines and which related specifically to the management of childhood constipation. This group included a consultant paediatric gastroenterologist, a paediatric pharmacist and nurses from the clinic. This group protocol was presented to the drug and therapeutics committee for approval.

VISUAL AIDS

A variety of visual aids should be available to help the children and their parents picture what is being described. As mentioned in earlier sections of this book, the Bristol Stool Form Chart, although designed for use with adults, has proved to be useful to ascertain what the child's stools are like. Clay models of stools are also available, which give a very graphic representation of stools. Other visual aids may include simple diagrams of the anatomy to help explain what happens and how the treatment works.

One of the best visual aids I have seen was demonstrated by its inventor at a meeting I attended with other colleagues who manage children with continence problems. These meeting are a good source of current information for health professionals and give a chance to network with others with similar interests. Dr Ken N. Wilkinson, Consultant Paediatrician at Airedale General Hospital, West Yorkshire gave a very entertaining presentation in May 2001, at which he demonstrated the visual aid he uses to explain constipation and soiling to children and parents. It is simple and available

---

Box 9.9   Points to remember

- A number of different visual aids can be used, but all must be acceptable to the professional and the client group
- Simplicity is the key to understanding

---

to anyone. He uses a 40 cm length of narrow (2 cm wide) tubigauze into which he inserts four chocolate-filled eggs to represent the 'poo'. The eggs are widely available, being made by several confectionery manufacturers. He holds one end of the tubigauze tightly closed to demonstrate an effective anus, and puts a kink in it to demonstrate the anorectal angle. He also shows how it can be used to demonstrate holding and the soiling which follows from the effect of holding on the anus, by pushing an egg to the end representing the anus and allowing it to keep the tubigauze open. This helps parents to understand why they can wipe and wipe, but there is always some staining on the tissue. I'm sure, with some imagination, other relevant uses for filled chocolate eggs and tubigauze will come to mind.

LANGUAGE

Although, as health professionals, we use a certain language because during our training this has gradually been taught to us along with all the other information, our patients do not necessarily have this knowledge. All manner of professional language can be used to exclude others not from the same group. If used with patients it can very effectively exclude them too. As adults, some parents will find 'health professional talk' difficult to translate, so children will find it almost impossible to understand. In cases such as these, where part of the management is aimed at helping children to take responsibility for their own condition, it helps if they do not feel excluded because the language used is inappropriate. So all embarrassment must be ignored and language that both the child and the parent can understand must be used. Whether talking about faeces ('poo') or stool softeners ('things that make the poo soft') or stimulant laxatives ('things that make the child poo'), families must be included.

Similarly, explanations of what will happen and how they are expected to react must be in words the families will understand, otherwise the health professional might as well speak Welsh or Latin.

Box 9.10 Points to remember

- One of the easiest ways to exclude a person is to use language they do not understand
- Use the words the child and the parent are familiar with
- All explanations should use words and terms that the child can understand; one of the aims of management is to get the child to take personal responsibility for the condition

---

WRITTEN INFORMATION

Information given to the child and the parent should be backed up with good quality, easily legible written information on a variety of topics. Explanations of laxatives, the bowel and how it works and why the soiling happens can all be included in a booklet to give to the child and the parent. Details about the treatment and how this will help the condition, and an indication of the length of time for which the treatment will continue for are all useful information for the family. The different types of laxatives should be explained, including how they work and why it is necessary to take more than one. A brief description of the different stages of treatment is useful, together with why it is important to complete each stage. There may be a need to have a different information sheet for different stages of treatment; the personal preference of local health professionals can be sought, as can local financial restrictions. Having individual sheets for distribution at varying stages of treatment may be preferred if they can be photocopied, because they can be given at the appropriate stage of management and if lost they are not so costly to replace. Although a booklet printed professionally may cover the whole treatment, it is very costly if it has to be replaced at each different stage because it has been mislaid by the child or parent.

Obviously, there needs to be negotiation between the health professional and management to agree on these issues prior to the clinic running. The information must be kept as simple as possible; do not forget the children and their parents will come from a wide range of backgrounds, so all levels must be catered for. It is helpful if there is space on the record sheet to write the health professional's name and a contact telephone number. Clayden (1996) suggests we should address some of the issues around this condition 'by supplying: detailed written information about the conditions for parents to use in explaining to family, friends, teachers and their own employers if necessary.'

Information for others involved in the care of this child can also be useful. The school nurse, health visitor, general practitioner, teaching staff, etc. may all need to know in varying degrees of detail about the child's care and how it affects what they do for the child. The health visitor will require details of the care being given and the progress being made; details of any stresses placed on the family and the possible impact on mothers' ability to care for her children may also be required. The school nurse needs similar information, and also details on special arrangements which may be needed in the school as the school nurse will often be the intermediary between school and other health professionals. The school will need basic information about the condition and how the management plan will impact on their care of the child during the day. If the general practitioner is to prescribe the laxative, professional courtesy suggests passing on information on the child's management. The regular letters from the health professional managing the child's condition, keeping the general practitioner up-to-date and requesting changes in medication, should also warn them that the laxatives will be required for many months, as most drug books warn against long-term use. It may be that it is decided to use standard letters which have spaces to be completed for the individual child with their particulars at an appointment. If secretarial support is available, it may be that individual letters can be written for each child. Local circumstances will, to some extent, dictate what format communication takes, but good practice suggests that it does take place in some form.

Box 9.11 Points to remember

- All explanations should be followed up with a written version
- Information leaflets or booklets should be designed to appeal to a wide audience and may vary from individual sheets about specific aspects of management to a booklet giving information about the whole treatment
- Contact information must be included upon the written information
- Written information on the progress of the child should be sent to the child's general practitioner and the person who made the referral
- Other professionals may need to be informed of the child's progress

---

DOCUMENTATION

As already discussed, all health professionals must ensure their record-keeping is at the highest standard. Using forms specifically designed for this condition is a first step, but all pages must be labelled with the patient's name and, as these children will be seen many times during their management, it is essential that records are kept securely when not in use. The papers, including reports, letters and results, should be filed in chronological order. Good practice suggests other aspects of record-keeping are important. The entries in the child's records should be clear and legible, a fact that over time has escaped many health professionals. They must also be relevant and honest, but factual and objective. The entries should also be consistent, concise, meaningful and jargon-free. As individuals have a right to be able to access their own health records now, they should also be understandable and contain no abbreviations. It is also suggested that they be completed in black ink and be signed and dated (the time of the appointment is also important) and up-to-date. The UKCC (1998) states on records:

There are a number of factors which contribute to effective record keeping. Patient and client records should:

- be factual, consistent and accurate
- be written as soon as possible after an event has occurred, providing current information on the care and condition of the patient or client
- be written clearly and in such a manner that the text cannot be erased
- be written in such a manner that any alterations or additions are dated, timed and signed in such a way that the original entry can still be read clearly
- be accurately dated, timed and signed, with the signature printed alongside the first entry
- not include abbreviations, jargon, meaningless phrases, irrelevant speculation and offensive subjective statements
- be readable on any photocopies.

In addition, records should:

- be written, wherever possible, with the involvement of the patient or client or their carer
- be written in terms that the patient can understand
- be consecutive
- identify problems that have arisen and the action taken to rectify them
- provide clear evidence of the care planned, the decisions made, the care delivered and the information shared.

As stated earlier, documentation of care given and the results of that care can help when reviewing a case to see what has been successful and what has not been. It is difficult to remember every detail of care given; for this reason accurate records are required—whether looking back for auditing purposes or to evaluate an aspect of care. It is also helpful to use past entries to remind both the child and the parent just how far they have come from the situation they described at their first appointment. All individuals will forget the details of what was happening 2 or 3 months ago if caught up in what is happening at present. If the child has been coming to a clinic for a year, their memories of the situation at the beginning will almost certainly have faded with the passage of time. Muir & Burnett (1999) also include record-keeping in their protocols; 'Recording clinical data to ensure both completeness of and consistency in the documentation of the child's progress.'

Earlier, it was mentioned that agreed plans should be documented so that on the child's return the health professional knows what he was to have completed. If the child or parent has not carried out what was requested of them and there is no suitable reason for this, one has to wonder if the management of this child is going to be successful. If there is failure to carry out agreed plans on a number of occasions, it is questionable whether the child and parent actually want success. In this case, it is appropriate to refer to a specialist who will examine motivation and encourage concordance with the treatment.

INVOLVING OTHERS

When managing any child with constipation and soiling, it is unlikely that the care will be delivered in isolation from others; in any child's life there are a number of professionals involved. Whether the others involved are restricted to the family health visitor and general practitioner, or whether they include school

---

Box 9.12 Points to remember

- All professionals should maintain adequate documentation
- There are legal requirements to keep records accurately
- Good record-keeping is essential for audit at a later date
- All records should be stored securely between appointments

nurse, school staff, family therapy nurse, playgroup or after school club workers, social workers and relatives, the aim should be the same, i.e. to involve them as much as the child and the parent wish. There may be some resistance from the child and the parent to involving others as they may want to keep the condition as secret as possible. Careful explanation and discussion about limiting those informed is vital. If they want secrecy, only those who really need to be told to allow the management to be carried out successfully should be involved. If regular toileting is part of the programme, anyone who can help to 'supervise' this needs to be included. If the child is recovering well and toileting once daily with no seepage, it is debatable if anyone other than those included for professional courtesy need to be informed.

Referrer

It is important, for professional courtesy and good practice, that when someone has referred a patient to another health professional they are informed of progress. It may be that the referrer can support the family in the management plan if they are aware of what is being suggested. Often they will have a better or longer relationship with the child and his parent than the health professional managing the constipation and soiling. This can be a valuable asset in the care of the child, if used wisely. They may be aware of previous problems, such as poor attendance at clinics, past child protection issues or previous attempts to manage the soiling. All this is important in the assessment of the child and the family. The referrer may be able to see the child and parent in between appointments to encourage concordance with the programme. The family may at first feel happier disclosing problems with the programme to the known professional and this, too, can be a useful addition to the management.

Health professionals

There are a number of professionals who may be involved in the management of a child. Some have already been mentioned; others may include a community paediatric nurse, if the child has special needs. A paediatric physiotherapist may also be involved if the child has special needs, but also if abdominal massage is offered as an adjunct to laxative treatment (see Chapter 10). An occupational therapist may also be invaluable for suggesting aids and appliances that help the child with special needs.

A valuable health professional to involve in difficult cases where there are questions around concordance with management is a family therapy nurse. These nurses usually have a qualification in mental health and can work with the family to look at blocks to treatment and encourage them to overcome the blocks and carry out the treatment. These nurses are, however, not a common resource and may not be available locally. If there is no similar resource available, there may be a paediatric nurse who has similar experience, or a child and family therapy unit that can advise other health professionals. A clinical psychologist could also be used in this situation, if there is such a service locally. Again, if the waiting list is too long, they may be willing to support other health professionals with suggestions about how to approach the case. Locally, I have always found them very helpful and supportive. Local resources will vary and it is an aspect of preparation for the clinic that the willingness of other services to assist be investigated.

Nursery or school staff

If the child attends a nursery or school, some involvement of the staff may be unavoidable, regardless of child and parental wishes. If they are having to support the child or help to clean up after an accident, it is vital that they are informed of what is happening and how best they can aid the management plan.

Good practice, as stated and discussed, has many aspects and to carry it out takes time, but it is time well spent. Think about how you would like to be treated yourself and what you would like in your records, and many will feel that what has been discussed is

---

Box 9.13 Points to remember

- Other health professionals may be more appropriate people to carry out certain aspects of management
- All relevant professionals should be informed how they can best support the child and parent in the management
- Investigate local resources: what does the physiotherapist in the area accept, what about clinical psychology—do they see children?
- Professional courtesy suggests certain other professionals should be enrolled into the plan

what they would like. This is the best measure of a professional's practice. Would you be happy if you were on the receiving end of your own care?

REFERENCES

Clayden 1996 A guide for good practice: childhood constipation. Ambulatory Child Health 1(5): 250–255
Department of Health 1998 A report on the supply and administration of medicines under group protocol. Review of Prescribing, Supply & Administration of Medicines. Department of Health, London
Department of Health 2001 Reference guide to consent for examination or treatment. Department of Health, London
Muir J, Burnett C 1999 Setting up a nurse-led clinic for intractable childhood constipation. British Journal of Community Nursing 4(8): 395–399
UKCC 1992 Code of Professional Conduct, UKCC, London
UKCC 1998 Guideline for records and record keeping. UKCC, London
UKCC 2000 Guidelines for the administration of medicines. UKCC, London
UKCC 2001 Supporting nurses, midwives and health visitors through lifelong learning. UKCC, London

10

Other options

Dietetics
Psychology
Physiotherapy
Continence advisors and
    nurse specialists

Complementary therapy
Occupational therapists
Aids

In this chapter, other aids and professionals and the contribution they can make to the management of children with constipation and soiling will be examined. Not all the professionals will be available in every area, so investigation of local resources is advised. Some professionals mentioned will almost certainly not be available within NHS provider units. Not only should the existence of the professionals mentioned be checked but it is also an idea to make contact with them to ascertain just exactly what they are prepared or able to offer in support for these children. In many cases it will be found that either there is no paediatric service or, if there is, the service is so stretched it can offer only support and advice to the professionals managing the children. Discuss the exact circumstance in which they could accept a referral from the service being set up. Do they only accept referrals from a doctor or only from health professionals or do they have an open referral system? Some services will accept self-referral from the parent and, in fact, will treat these cases as more urgent than referrals from other professionals. The premise behind this is that if parents are going to the trouble to contact the service, their need must be great. Make a note of the details gained during these discussions and keep these as up-to-date as possible; perhaps annual contact with the services may give information on any changes in the service. Some services will be more approachable than others and some will be more than willing to help; others, because of constraints placed upon them by the local employer, will be wishing to help but unable to do so at present. All the information gathered will be useful as it gives a starting point for the professional who wishes to manage the children with constipation and soiling. A quick reference guide to inform the professional exactly who is able to accept referrals, and from whom, and what services they can offer to the client group may prove very valuable when a complex case occurs.

In the pages that follow are some suggestions of the type of help different services can offer in relation to the management of children with this distressing condition. As stated, some will be available to you, others may not; those that are available may not be able to offer exactly the service that is described. All health service providers have different views of what is an acceptable level of service, and in the absence of another service requiring support from a potentially small team it is difficult to anticipate all the demands that will be placed on a particular area of practice.

DIETETICS

Many health service providers employ at least one dietician to advise the population they serve on specific areas of dietary health. Some will have a dietician dedicated to advising children on dietary matters. A number will hold a caseload of children who need advice and will, if time allows, see children referred from other health professionals for conditions such as constipation. In many areas, the team is small and the need great so they will teach other health professionals about the basics of good dietary intake and support them with information to enable the health professional to give dietary advice. If these sessions are available locally, take advantage of them as they can prove to be very useful when advising clients on dietary matters. This means their more expert knowledge is reserved for the more complicated cases that really need a dietician. This represents effective use of resources, but is not helpful if a new service is being considered and support is not available from dieticians as required. Some dieticians are happy to become involved in teaching on specific subjects such as the need for a high-fibre diet. They may be willing to teach on dietary issues if ever a local in-service training day on constipation and soiling is considered. They will also provide information leaflets and food suggestions on how to disguise fibre within a diet to tempt children to eat it. A nursing colleague of mine told me if they had mashed potatoes at home she always put in turnips as they are the same colour and it added to the vegetables the children were eating. However, dieticians tend not to give advice in terms of the number of grams of fibre a day a child should eat. Because they work within the limits and recommendations of British advisory panels which give these as percentages of total intake, this is the format they use. At present, it is around 30% of total intake.

If applying for funding to start a clinic, ask for some time for a dietician to be included in the professionals staffing the service. Even if they are not appointed full-time, the advice they can offer both to families and health professionals is invaluable. If they were available for only one session each week, the service they could offer clients would still be tremendous. If a dietician cannot be present, make sure the resources available to staff regarding diet and particularly high fibre are of excellent quality. The local dietetics department should be able to advise on this and can supply the leaflets required.

PSYCHOLOGY

Support for the psychological aspects of management of children with constipation and soiling can be found from a variety of different services, some of which have been mentioned earlier in this book. Briefly, these services will include clinical psychology, child and family therapy or child and adolescent mental health services and nurse specialists—family therapy. The support of a professional with training in mental health or psychology can be utilised in a number of ways. The aspects of management that they can be invaluable with are in supporting compliance or concordance with the management plan by the child and family, behaviour management techniques and rewards. Equally importantly, they can help the health professional and the child's parent to understand the concept of externalisation in relation to the condition, if this approach is considered a suitable adjunct to therapy for an individual child and family. This is a complex psychological theory but, in brief, it means that instead of blaming the child or others for the 'poo' escaping and causing all the problems, the 'poo' is blamed and the child and other members of the family are recruited to try to beat the 'poo'. The 'poo' is beaten when it stops escaping and causing, for example, family arguments or the child to hide his underwear. Other helpers may be recruited into the fight against the 'poo', including the medicines prescribed and a timer to time visits to the toilet. There is a story book called *"Beating Sneaky Poo"* written by Terry Heins and Karen Ritchie and illustrated by Geoff Pryor and Quantum. It is an Australian book and is well received by children with the condition of constipation and soiling. The book gives 'sneaky poo' a personality which some psychologists feel is inappropriate but the personalities of the helpers in the fight against 'sneaky poo' are also forceful and equal to the fight. Of course, one problem with externalising the 'poo' is that the family could be alienated. The process of externalising is usually started from the first appointment, before the family's likes and dislikes are well established. The age range that this can be used for is limited too. Talking to a 13- or 14-year-old about 'sneaky poo' is not appropriate; they are too mature to appreciate this approach. Very young children may become frightened of the 'sneaky poo' if the story around it is not carefully controlled, as the 'poo' can take on monster-like features. If this becomes the case, the child may develop a fear of visiting the toilet where other 'sneaky poos' live and he may increase the retention in a bid to prevent the 'monster sneaky poo' escaping, which will then compound his original problem. The approach should be used with care and each family assessed individually so that it suits their circumstances. Although there are steps within the process, it is not something that can be rigidly applied to every family. Children with little verbal communication or perception problems, such as children suffering from the autistic spectrum disorders, may find externalising very difficult. Lack of imagination results in an inability to perceive the 'poo' as something that requires defeating.

Helping to support the family to improve concordance with the management plan can be a vital aspect of the treatment for some families. If there are various social problems or the family life is chaotic, the support that can be gained from family therapy nurses or mental health-trained nurses can prove invaluable. The nurses have the expert knowledge to help families cope with the demands that a management plan for this type of condition requires. If the nurse has the right type of job description, their support can be delivered both in hospital but more importantly at the child's home. Being able to visit the home gives a much better picture of the social constraints on the family, and the environment in which the child and parent are trying to carry out the management.

Colleagues have given appalling descriptions of the bathrooms in some homes which would give few people the confidence to use them. For a child learning to use a toilet properly for the first time, the bathroom plays a major role, as described earlier in this book. When supporting families with concordance, one aspect used is to help them make a choice about the treatment by looking at what happens at present when the soiling occurs. This may include dirty pants, mum being cross and the child being teased at school and feeling bad. The medicine will hopefully give the opposite of these bad feelings and the child will therefore choose to take the medicines as prescribed. The family will also need help to antici-pate failure and to plan what they can do when it happens. Understanding the basics of behaviour management is important for any professional who wishes to treat children with any condi-tion requiring a change from undesirable to desirable behaviour, such as soiling. Psychological research has given the background knowledge for behaviour management which plays an important role in the management of these children. The appropriate use of rewards and the theory behind the techniques used in manage-ment can be utilised by any professional with basic knowledge, but more complex cases benefit from the enhanced and expert help of those with psychological training. For those families where there are extra difficulties, the professional advice and support of either a clinical psychologist or mental health-trained nurse can make all the difference to the success of a management plan. In cases where there is now a degree of encopresis involved, a referral to one of these experts may pay dividends for the family as well as the pro-fessional.

PHYSIOTHERAPY

Physiotherapists can be especially valuable when managing cases involving children with special needs. They can give exercises and tips for helping the children to sit upright when on the toilet. Their skills can be used for other aspects of treat-ment too.

De Paepe et al (2000) looked at the role of pelvic floor exercis-es in the treatment of children with enuresis and constipation and soiling with great success. The children involved in their study were all under 5 years of age and 16 had continence prob-lems:

. . . (three diurnal, two nocturnal and 11 both diurnal and nocturnal). In the group with incontinence problems, recurrent UTIs occurred in seven girls, perineal pain in two children, vaginal irritation in five girls and obstipation (a term used for constipation) in four children. Four children were completely dry but complained of other urological symptoms . . .

The children were taught pelvic floor exercises. Because a potty was found to give a poor position for defecation, as the extra depth to the squat encouraged the child to strain, parents were asked to ensure that the child sat on a normal toilet with 'a toilet-reducer and a small bench or support under the feet.' They also completed a voiding and drinking chart, and those with urody-namically confirmed detrusor instability were treated with oxy-butinin; those with recurrent UTIs had prophylactic antibiotics and the children with constipation were given 'drugs to relieve the impaction.' The results were impressive as 'Whereas only four children were completely dry before treatment, 17 were com-pletely dry afterward . . . in five of eight children the obstipation resolved.'

As seen in Chapter 2, the pelvic floor plays an important role in maintaining continence and in the process of defecation, and children can be taught how to use the muscles to relax to allow the faecal mass to pass and then to tighten the muscle afterwards to keep the sphincter closed. Physiotherapists are expert at mus-cle exercises and their role in the teaching of pelvic floor exercis-es after assessment should not be overlooked. Of course, if they are already too busy and unable to accept children for this type of treatment, it may be that they are able to train other professionals to teach children pelvic floor exercises.

Another role for physiotherapists is in carrying out and teach-ing abdominal massage to help increase colonic motility. Chiarelli & Markwell (1992) advocate that adults suffering from constipa-tion should practice it on themselves and give instructions as fol-lows:

Lie with the upper half of your body supported by pillows. Place a pillow beneath your knees so that they are supported in a slightly bent position.
Your hands should be warm, and their pressure should be firm. You will probably be able to feel the bowel contents if you're constipated. Remember that the colon begins in the lower right hand corner of the abdomen. This is where the massage should begin.

- Your abdomen should be bare. If you feel cold, cover yourself with a rug or blanket
- Using a firm, gentle pressure, make large stroking movements up your right side, across under the rib cage and down the left side of your abdomen. This is the direction of movement along the colon. These large movements are called effleurage
- These stroking movements can be followed by small circular movements, always following the same direction as the bowel contents. Repeat each small circular movement about six times before changing your hand position
- Continue the massage for about 10 minutes or until your hands get tired

This massage should be a pleasant experience. If you feel any discomfort, stop immediately.

A physiotherapist will have a slightly more refined approach to abdominal massage, which is highly effective. As with all therapies outside a nurse's basic training, it is important that unless a specific training course has been attended it is advised that this be left to the professional most able to give it. The physiotherapist can give training to the parent to carry out the massage at home as an adjunct to laxative therapy. Bland massage oil such as that available from such outlets as 'The Body Shop' are useful for this type of treatment. Massage, if properly carried out, can be effective and can also strengthen the bond between the parent and child. Having observed a demonstration of abdominal massage carried out by a physiotherapist on a colleague, I can recommend this treatment and feel that, if possible, it should be included in the range of treatments offered to children and parents. The dramatic result in the colleague was certainly enough to convert those present to believe in the benefit of this treatment to the children being managed. As stated, it is not intended to replace the laxative therapy but to be in addition to it. It is particularly useful for children with special needs, but can be effective for all. When demonstrating the procedure, it is vital that there are no overtones of sexual intent with it, so always use the term abdominal massage, not just massage, a professional attitude and bland oil. One has to be careful when talking about many aspects of this condition not to imply a sexual overtone to the treatments suggested.

CONTINENCE ADVISORS & NURSE SPECIALISTS

Some areas have a continence advisor who has experience and expertise in treating children; some areas have not. Other areas employ a paediatric or children's continence advisor, and yet others use nurses from specialities such as school nursing to run clinics for enuretic children. Whatever happens locally, there is some value in making contact with the continence advisor or equivalent. As each health service provider has a duty to provide a continence service of some type, there should be someone who has this role. Each will have a particular area of expertise and all will have access to resources that may not be available to other staff. Some will control the use of continence aids that may be required, including perhaps enuresis alarms, some will have budgetary responsibility for continence. Even if the continence advisor in the local area does not include children in the remit of their service, contact them. They will have detailed knowledge about constipation and can offer advice on assessment tools or on running clinics, where to obtain help, company details for literature to be given to clients, etc. They can often provide a sounding board to listen to ideas about protocols or referrals systems as they will have carried out a similar process. If the protocols they have in place are acceptable with minor adjustment, use them; why reinvent the wheel?

The continence advisor who includes children in her client group can prove to be a double-edged sword if you wish to manage children with this condition. On the one hand, they can offer expert support and advice but on the other, they may have a remit which suggests all children should be referred to their care. Many are happy to see straightforward cases managed locally while concentrating their own expertise on the more complex cases deserving of their time. Local nurse specialists may also have a remit that suggests that no other nurses locally will gain any experience or expertise in treating children with continence problems. While this results in only those with, hopefully up-to-date, knowledge managing children with constipation and soiling and who are, hopefully, enthusiastic about the management, it also results in other staff being unable to test their own enthusiasm for the management of these conditions. There should, therefore, be built into any system employing this type of staff the opportunity for other staff to work alongside the specialists.

COMPLEMENTARY THERAPY

There is a wide range of alternative or complementary therapies that can be utilised in the management of children with constipation and soiling. Some complementary therapies are available within the NHS now, but others are still not available and are unlikely to be for some time. As with all treatments that are not within practitioners' own experience or knowledge, any complementary therapies should be carried out by recognised practitioners. There is now a register of complementary therapists which will include only reputable practitioners. However, not all complementary therapies are included on the register. Professional judgement should be used when recommending any of these therapies and specific practitioners.

Aromatherapy. Therapies such as aromatherapy have been used for thousands of years and by a wide range of people to help in a myriad of situations from relaxation to curing headaches. Aromatherapy uses essential oils from flowers, herbs and spices, and the oils can be used topically or as an inhalation. Care should be taken when using any essential oils on children as they can be absorbed through the skin and some can cause problems once absorbed. Certain herbs and flowers are known to help with digestive problems and would be used by a practitioner to ease constipation. If abdominal massage is being used it might be used in conjunction with aromatherapy.

Herbalism as its name suggests, uses herbs and plants to treat many different symptoms of illnesses. This form of medicine predates conventional medicine by centuries. In fact, throughout this book mention has been made of the usefulness of this more natural medicine. Liquorice has been known since time immemorial to ease constipation, as has rhubarb. Senna is also a plant derivative which is still used today as it is so effective. Other seeds and herbs are known to reduce flatulence and can be added to meals to ease this embarrassing problem. There are many books available that discuss using different plants and herbs to treat minor ailments. If planning to use this type of information, ensure it is from a reputable source.

Reflexology has also been practised for thousands of years in a number of different cultures. In this therapy, different areas of the hands and feet are thought to represent different organs or areas of the body. By applying pressure to the relevant area of the hand or foot, it stimulates the organ represented and improves the blood flow to the organ. The therapy should be applied on several occasions each day to the relevant area. The fleshy area at the base of the thumb is supposed to represent the colon, as is the arch of the foot.

Acupuncture is perhaps one of the better known of the complementary or alternative therapies. This ancient Chinese art has been used for centuries. Again, different organs are represented by areas elsewhere on the body and at these points fine sterile needles are inserted and either moved gently or sometimes heated by burning a substance on the end of the needle. This healing art form should be obtained only from specially trained practitioners with an excellent reputation and an entry on the register mentioned.

Shiatsu has over time developed from acupuncture, as similar points on the body are used but instead of inserting needles to the points, pressure is applied. In the western world, perhaps the most well-known application of shiatsu is in travel bands or morning sickness bands—these prevent nausea by applying pressure to a point on the inner wrist. They are comprised of a bracelet of elastic material with a 'button' that is placed by the wearer over the appropriate point on the wrist. I have certainly used these with good effects for myself and my son during long car journeys.

Homeopathy treats illnesses with a small dose of a substance that produces the same ailment. This is then supposed to stimulate the body to overcome the ailment and heal itself. Each individual would be given a different combination of substances for the same ailment, depending upon the patient and the practitioner. There have been many well-known proponents of homeopathy.

Massage too may be considered an alternative therapy. It has been used for many hundreds of years to ease some ailments and to treat aches and pains. By massaging areas slowly, muscle tension is relieved and blood supply and lymphatic drainage is improved. (Adapted from Getliffe & Dolman 1997.)

OCCUPATIONAL THERAPISTS

This profession assesses a patient's need for various aids and adaptations to allow them to live as normal a life as possible. It may be the need for a wheelchair or something as simple as a device to aid in opening jars. Children with special needs will often be known by the local occupational therapy department. Many aspects of their life may already be being helped by aids and adaptations suggested by their Occupational Therapist (OT). If there appear to be specific issues around toiletting the child, it is well worth bringing them in to assess the situation and organise the appropriate solution to the problem. If the problem is at school as well as at home, there should be a system in place to allow the child to have similar aids at school and home to make the problem easier. Most children do not have to transport all their special requirements to and from school every day.

AIDS

There are a number of aids that can be useful when managing children with chronic constipation and soiling. Some have been designed specifically to help a child's understanding of the process of defecation; others are designed to help the professional. Whatever aids you find useful should be contained in your 'clinic kit'. The *Bonner Blower* was designed by a continence advisor from Luton. This device is for children and helps them to understand that although they should contract abdominal and thoracic muscles during defecation, they should continue to exhale. It is similar to a party blower, but does not extend. It makes what is for children a satisfying noise. This is a useful addition to the 'kit' described earlier, together with details of how it can be obtained if you feel it is worthwhile.

Many of the other aids have been described earlier in the text. Good quality aids can be difficult to obtain, but if found it is worth getting them at the time. Some funding, if available, to buy small aids and rewards for children successfully completing their management plans is very useful. The cost can be quite small, but exploration of your employing authority's policy on this issue should be carried out before going ahead to start a fund.

This text has covered all aspects of managing children with chronic constipation and soiling. Some points covered are well known, others less well known; all have a degree of importance in contributing to the understanding of this distressing condition from which children can suffer. If you have read this far you are probably already converted and realise the benefit of managing the children effectively. Managing children with constipation and soiling can be rewarding, though at times disheartening. If properly planned, a clinic for these children can be a good place for the families to visit. If this book has helped to stimulate an interest in managing these children it has done its job!

REFERENCES

Chiarelli P, Markwell S 1992 Let's get thing's moving, overcoming constipation. NSW Gore & Osment Publications, Woollahra

De Paepe H, Renson C, Van Laecke E, Raes A, Vande Walle J, Hoebeke P 2000 Pelvic floor therapy and toilet training in young children with dysfunctional voiding and obstipation. BJU International 85(7): 889–893

Getliffe K, Dolman M 1997 Promoting continence: a clinical and research resource. Baillière Tindall, London

Heins T, Ritchie K 1985 Beating Sneaky Poo: ideas for faecal soiling. Canberra Publishing & Printing Company, Canberra

Index